Ayurveda

A Quick Reference Handbook

DR. MANISHA KSHIRSAGAR BAMS, DY&A (AYURVEDA, INDIA)

ANA CRISTINA R. MAGNO, BA, MS, AWC, CMT

LOTUS
PRESS

P.O. Box 325
Twin Lakes, WI 53181 USA

Disclaimer
Ayurveda: A Quick Reference Handbook is a basic introduction to the vast subject of Ayurveda.

The authors and publisher assume no responsibility or liability for the reader's actions or interpretation of the material found in this book. The reader should consult a health care certified professional for guidance in the use of techniques, treatments and herbs or any subject mentioned in this book.

Color version ISBN: 978-0-9406-7697-8
B&W version ISBN: 978-0-9406-7695-4

Library of Congress Control Number: 2011929095

Printed in the United States of America

LOTUS
PRESS

Published by:
Lotus Press, P.O. Box 325, Twin Lakes, WI 53181 USA
web: www.lotuspress.com
Email: lotuspress@lotuspress.com
800.824.6396

acknowledgments

So many hearts and hands have helped us write this book. Our deepest gratitude goes out to all the past and modern day sages who have illuminated the timeless wisdom throughout the ages.

From Manisha Kshirsagar

First and foremost, I would like to express my heartfelt thanks to my dear parents and my brother, who instilled in me the valuable life lessons of patience, contentment, and flexibility. Sincere thanks to my wonderful in-laws, who encouraged me to travel abroad and find my wings. My beloved husband Dr. Suhas, who like "Prana" has enriched my life in every possible way. My loving kids, Manas and Sanika, their unconditional love has always been a foundation of my life.

My deep gratitude to Maharishi Mahesh Yogi for giving me the direct experience and understanding of the most fundamental nature of reality. I feel deeply blessed.

From Ana Cristina R. Magno

My earnest gratitude and thanks to my mother for her kindness, love and endless support throughout my life in my endeavours.

My family for their devotion, love, support, generosity and belief in my dreams, every step of the way.

Many thanks to my personal friends, and you know who you are, for sharing their professional expertise, their consistent feedback, encouragement and praise.

Sincere thanks to Dr. Suhas, for sharing his wisdom, insight and continuous support throughout this project.

Our gratitude goes to all our teachers and colleagues. We deeply appreciate the help from Dr. David Frawley, who recommended us to Lotus Press. His words of encouragement and wholehearted endorsement has brought the book to fruition.

Thanks to Dr. Vasant Lad, who is a true inspiration, and his foreword in this book.

Dr. David Simon and Dr. Deepak Chopra are true modern day sages, who have helped Ayurveda and Yoga regain its ancient glory. We deeply admire their support.

Our thanks to Cynthia Copple for her endorsement, as well as her extraordinary and profound insights.

Lastly, many thanks to Santosh and Shanta Krinsky from Lotus Press, who appreciated our efforts and decided to publish this book.

contents

foreword

Ayurveda is an ancient Vedic system of healing. It is timeless wisdom brought to the practical level in our day-to-day life. According to this system, every individual is indivisible, undivided, complete, a total unique expression of cosmic consciousness. We are individual, but we are not yet undivided because individual means total, and we are fragmented, broken up. Therefore, people in the world don't really know who they are. They don't know their constitution, their prakruti and vikruti, current state. People eat and live according to their moods and their emotions and, by doing this, they create an internal imbalance of vata, pitta, and kapha that may manifest into psychosomatic disorders.

Vata, pitta, and kapha are the basic three organizations of the human body and they govern our unique psycho physiology. Our unique nature is prakruti and prakruti is constantly bombarded by seasonal changes, dietary fluctuations, emotional upsets, job changes, and environmental differences. These variations cause the doshas to change and create a unique syndrome of imbalance known as vikruti, the altered state of the dosha.

Ayurvedic science is based on a great foundation, a profound philosophy, and practical clinical observation. It also has a unique therapeutic value, including panchakarma (detoxification program), rasayana (rejuvenation program), and dinacharya (diet and lifestyle program). In this sense, it is the science of longevity of life.

Dr. Manisha Kshirsagar and Ana Cristina R. Magno have put this wonderful, vast science into a beautiful tabular form with explanations. It will become easier for the beginner to memorize these facts of the basic principles of Ayurveda, such as the number of subdoshas, the upadhatus, how we can see the effect of agnis and the bhuta agnis as well as the dhatu agni. This book makes it very clear and simple for students, practitioners, and Ayurvedic newcomers to memorize this factual knowledge. I hope this book will definitely inspire the students, practitioners, and beginners.

Dr. Manisha Kshirsagar and Ana Cristina R. Magno have wonderfully brought this ageless wisdom into daily practical living through this book.

Thank you and I bless this book with my love and compassion.

Dr. Vasant Lad
Director of Ayurveda Institute of New Mexico
March 2011

introduction

Ayurveda: a Quick Reference Handbook is a simple, clear and practical guide to the fundamentals of Ayurvedic medicine both for self-care and for clinical application. The books' well-designed format easily lends itself as a teaching manual for this otherwise difficult subject, being structured like a comprehensive power point presentation. It presents the main teachings of Ayurveda derived from classical texts in a concise and almost sutra like manner. Its tabular format can help both students and laypeople understand the key concepts and practices of Ayurveda quickly and easily commit them to memory.

In addition, the book presents Ayurveda along with its greater Vedic and Yogic connections. Its study of Yoga is also clear and comprehensive, including all aspects of classical Yoga from asana to meditation. The book introduces the reader to the entire spectrum of Vedic sciences that Ayurveda has always been closely connected to, most notably Vedic astrology and Vastu, for showing how the forces of time and space impact our health, well-being and consciousness as a whole.

Ayurveda: a Quick Reference Handbook is an important pocket reference for anyone interested in Ayurveda, Yoga or the Vedic sciences in general. It condenses in a few pages what other books labor to explain in many chapters. As such, the book complements other studies of Ayurveda, and makes them more accessible as well.

Dr. Manisha Kshirsagar and Cristina Magno have performed an important service in presenting Ayurveda in a lucid and fresh manner, which will aid in the proper understanding and dissemination of Ayurveda's important teachings that can bring health and happiness to all. As Ayurveda continues to become more popular worldwide, the book should continue to be relevant for years to come.

Dr. David Frawley
Director of the American Institute of Vedic Studies
Author of more than thirty published books and several courses in Ayurveda, Yoga and the Vedic Sciences available in over fifteen different languages.

Ayurveda

Ayurveda principles

WHAT IS THE MEANING OF AYURVEDA?

Ayurveda is a Sanskrit term, made up of two words "ayu" and "veda". Ayu means life and Veda means science or knowledge. It is translated as Science of Life.

It is one of the most ancient and comprehensive medical sciences of the world. Ayurveda is a science for your mind, body and spirit. It is a consciousness-based approach to health that brings harmony and balance in all areas of your life.

WHAT IS THE ORIGIN OF AYURVEDA?

Ayurveda has its origins in the Veda, the oldest and richest text form of wisdom on spiritual knowledge on the planet. Ayurveda is considered a part of one of the four Vedas – Atharva-veda, that originated in India fi ve to six thousand years ago.

WHAT IS THE UNIQUENESS OF AYURVEDA?

Prevent, heal and preserve life.

Ayurveda is based upon the laws of nature. It is a holistic and natural medicine considered "Yatha Pinde tatha Bramhande", which means "as is the Macrocosm, so is the Microcosm". The relationship between the human being and the universe is intrinsic and cannot be separated. Ayurveda emphasizes balance and harmony with help from nature itself. This dynamic balance needs to be achieved in all aspects of a person's life: physical, biochemical, intellectual, emotional, behavioral, spiritual, familial, social, environmental and universal. Thus, Ayurveda treats the individual with all three dimensions: body, mind, and spirit, placing more emphasis on the prevention of diseases with the help of diet, daily routines, and seasonal routines. It also deals with diseases, their diagnosis and treatments with a unique approach toward purification and rejuvenation.

WHAT ARE THE BASIC PRINCIPLES?

Ayurveda believes that the universe is made up of five elements: air, fire, water, earth, and ether. These elements are the building blocks for the universe as well as for humans. From the combination of these elements, three "doshas" or energies: Vata, Pitta and Kapha are originated. Every person has a unique constitution that depends upon the right balance of the three doshas ("tridoshas"). Ayurveda suggests specific lifestyle and dietary changes to help individuals in balancing the doshas. According to Ayurveda, the definition of a healthy person is "one who has balanced doshas, balanced agni, properly formed dhatus, proper elimination of waste products, all bodily functions are proper, and whose soul, mind, and all five senses are in bliss".

ashtanga ayurveda

EIGHT FOLD CLASSIFICATION
Ayurveda is divided into eight branches of treatment

BRANCHES		BRANCHES	
Kaya Chikitsa	Internal medicine	Agada Tantra	Toxicology
Shalya Tantra	Surgery	Bhuta Vidya	Psychiatry
Shalakya Tantra	Ear, nose, throat, eye diseases	Rasayana	Rejuvenation therapy
Kaumarbhritya	Pediatrics	Vajeekarana	Aphrodisiac therapy

panchamahabhutas

THE FIVE ELEMENTS
Pancha–five | Mahabhutas–elements

The five basic main elements in nature are:

Akasha | Ether   Vayu | Air   Teja | Fire   Aap | Water   Prithvi | Earth

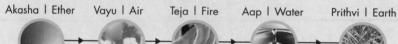

MAHABHUTAS	QUALITIES
Akasha	Ether	Subtle, soft, clear, smooth, expanding
Vayu	Air	Rough, dry, light, cold, mobile
Teja	Fire	Hot, sharp
Aap	Water	Flowing, wet, dull, soft, cloudy
Prithvi	Earth	Gross, heavy, static, hard, dense

The senses and the elements

MAHABHUTAS, SENSE ORGANS, MOTOR ORGANS AND TANMATRAS

MAHABHUTAS	SENSE ORGANS	MOTOR ORGANS	TANMATRAS
Akasha	Ether	Ear	Vocal Chords	Shabda (Sound)
Vayu	Air	Skin	Hands	Sparsha (Touch)
Teja	Fire	Eye	Feet	Rupa (Sight)
Aap	Water	Tongue	Genitals	Rasa (Taste)
Prithvi	Earth	Nose	Anus	Gandha (Smell)

doshas

DOSHAS OR THE THEORY OF BIO-ENERGIES
Vata, Pitta, Kapha

According to Ayurveda, the five main elements, or Panchamahabhutas, when combined give rise to doshas. These three doshas are found in our body. They are responsible for all biological and psychological functions, and they are present in all of us.

The three doshas are Vata, Pitta and Kapha, and each one is composed of two main elements. Vata dosha is a combination of space and air. It is responsible for every movement in the body, such as impulses, circulation, respiration, and elimination. Pitta dosha is a combination of fire and water. These two opposite forces represent transformation. Pitta governs heat, metabolism, temperature, transformation, and all chemical reactions. Kapha dosha is a combination of water and earth. It is responsible for growth, protection, lubrication, and sustenance.

These doshas, when stable, will generate a healthy constitution.

With the five elements and three doshas, Ayurveda determines the basic nature of an individual and prescribes a distinctive treatment plan according to their unique constitution.

VATA

The energy of action, transportation, and movement.

Composition   Ether + Air
Qualities   Light, dry, cold, rough, subtle and mobile

PITTA

The energy of transformation, conversion, and metabolism.

Composition   Fire + Water
Qualities   Light, hot, sharp, oily, mobile, liquid

KAPHA

The energy of construction, lubrication, and nourishment.

Composition   Water + Earth
Qualities   Heavy, cold, moist, dull, soft, sticky and static

subdoshas

VATA SUBDOSHAS
Prana, Udana, Samana, Apana, Vyana

SUBDOSHA	LOCATION (primary)	MOVEMENT
Prana	Head, brain	Downward, inward
Udana	Chest, throat	Upward
Samana	Small intestine	Periphery to center
Apana	Colon, pelvic area	Downward, outward
Vyana	Heart, whole body	Center to periphery

SUBDOSHA	
Prana	**Action** Controls the other vayus, inhalation, the senses, mind, consciousness. **Imbalance** Confusion, anxiety, fear, insomnia, debilitated senses.
Udana	**Action** Controls exhalation, speech, memory recollection, the upward movements of the body. **Imbalance** Problems with speech and throat, lung disorders, weak memory, indecisiveness.
Samana	**Action** Controls digestion, balances bodily systems. It is the meeting point of prana and apana. **Imbalance** Indigestion, constipation, loss of appetite, poor absorption.
Apana	**Action** Controls elimination, sexual function, menstruation, downward movement in the body. **Imbalance** Constipation, diarrhea, pain during menses, hormonal imbalance, urinary problems.
Vyana	**Action** Controls the heart, circulation of blood, muscular and joint movements. **Imbalance** Poor circulation, heart palpitations, anxiety, motor reflex problems.

subdoshas

PITTA SUBDOSHAS
Sadhaka, Alochaka, Pachaka, Ranjaka, Bhrajaka

SUBDOSHA	LOCATION (primary)	MAIN FUNCTIONS
Sadhaka	Brain, heart	Thinking, emotions, understanding
Alochaka	Eyes	Visual perception
Pachaka	Small intestine, stomach	Digestion of food
Ranjaka	Liver, spleen, small intestine	Gives color to blood
Bhrajaka	Skin	Skin color and texture

SUBDOSHA		
Sadhaka	**Action**	Responsible for thoughts, knowledge, discernment, awareness.
	Imbalance	Anger, jealousy, hesitation.
Alochaka	**Action**	Responsible for optical perception.
	Imbalance	Disorders of the eye.
Pachaka	**Action**	Responsible for digestion, absorption of food.
	Imbalance	Indigestion, hyperacidity, gastritis, nausea, peptic ulcers.
Ranjaka	**Action**	Responsible for blood's color, tissues, urine, feces.
	Imbalance	Hepatitis, jaundice, anemia, bleeding disorders.
Bhrajaka	**Action**	Responsible for skin pigmentation, luster.
	Imbalance	Skin conditions, eczema, dermatitis, psoriasis, moles, melanoma, hives.

subdoshas

KAPHA SUBDOSHAS
Tarpaka, Avalambaka, Kledaka, Bodhaka, Shleshaka

SUBDOSHA	LOCATION (primary)	MAIN FUNCTIONS
Tarpaka	Brain, cerebrospinal fluid	Supports subliminal thinking and memory
Avalambaka	Thoracic cavity	Supports all Kapha systems
Kledaka	Stomach (upper part)	Gastric secretion, digestion and absorption
Bodhaka	Mouth, tongue	Moistens oral cavity
Shleshaka	Joints	Lubricates joints, nourishes bones

SUBDOSHA	
Tarpaka	**Action** Protects nervous system, nourishes brain and nervous cells. **Imbalance** Lack of clarity and comprehension, loss of memory.
Avalambaka	**Action** Lubricates and nourishes lungs, heart, spine. **Imbalance** Asthma, bronchitis, pleurisy, emphysema.
Kledaka	**Action** Liquefies food in the stomach, nourishes and preserves the stomach lining. **Imbalance** Gastritis, indigestion, peptic ulcers.
Bodhaka	**Action** Controls taste, saliva, speech, lubricates mucus membrane. **Imbalance** Receding gum, plaque, loss of taste, congestion in the throat area.
Shleshaka	**Action** Lubricates joints in the body, nourishes the bones and cartilages. **Imbalance** Rheumatoid arthritis, swollen joints.

gunas

WHAT ARE QUALITIES OR ATTRIBUTES?

Qualities or attributes are a fundamental principle in Ayurveda. There are 20 qualities (pair of opposites) and each one associates with a different dosha. Each attribute is used to aid in finding what helps or aggravates a dosha.

ATTRIBUTES	ACTIONS	EXAMPLES
Heavy I Guru	Nourishing	Ashvagandha, banana, cheese, milk, wheat
Light I Laghu	Lightening	Black pepper, popcorn, puffed rice, lemon
Cold I Sheeta	Cooling	Neem, sandalwood
Hot I Ushna	Heating	Black pepper, ginger
Unctuous I Snigdha	Moistening	Ghee, oil, fat
Dry I Ruksha	Drying/Dehydrating	Haritaki, pepper, popcorn
Slow I Manda	Sluggish/Slowing	Milk, shatavari, squash
Sharp I Teekshna	Penetrating	Chilli pepper, mustard
Smooth I Slakshna	Oleating	Amalaki, grapes, shatavari
Rough I Khara	Roughening	Beans, calamus, raw vegetables
Dense I Sandra	Bulk promoting	Ashvagandha, butter, ghee
Liquid I Drava	Liquefying	Milk, water
Soft I Mrudu	Softening	Butter, ghee, lotus
Hard I Kathina	Hardening	Coral
Static I Sthira	Stabilizing	Chitrak, salt, turmeric
Mobile I Chala	Mobilizing	Haritaki, lemonade, senna
Gross I Sthula	Tonifying	Butter, cheese, meat
Subtle I Sookshma	Quick Spreading	Alcohol, black pepper, long pepper
Cloudy I Picchil	Adhering	Basil, flax seeds, psyllium husk
Clear I Vishada	Cleansing	Chitrak, salt, turmeric

gunas

THE TATTVAS AND THE TRIDOSHAS

ATTRIBUTES	VATA	PITTA	KAPHA	ATTRIBUTES	VATA	PITTA	KAPHA
Heavy | Guru	↓	↓	↑	Dense | Sandra	↓	↓	↑
Light | Laghu	↑	↑	↓	Liquid | Drava	↑	↑	↓
Cold | Sheeta	↑	↓	↑	Soft | Mrudu	↓	↑	↑
Hot | Ushna	↓	↑	↓	Hard | Kathina	↑	↓	↓
Oily | Snigdha	↓	↑	↑	Stable | Sthira	↓	↓	↑
Dry | Ruksha	↑	↓	↓	Mobile | Chala	↑	↑	↓
Dull | Manda	↓	↓	↑	Gross | Sthoola	↓	↓	↑
Sharp | Teekshna	↑	↑	↓	Subtle | Sookshma	↑	↑	↓
Smooth | Shlakshna	↓	↓	↑	Cloudy | Picchil	↓	↓	↑
Rough | Khara	↑	↓	↓	Clear | Vishada	↑	↑	↓

prakriti

PHYSICAL CONSTITUTION

According to Ayurveda, prakriti or physical constitution plays great significance in comprehending an individual's mental and physical characteristics. Finding the adequate prakriti is critical in order to determine the course of treatment for the individual. There are different types of prakriti.

TYPE	DESCRIPTION
V, P, K	Predominant in one dosha
VP, PV, PK, KP, KV, VK	Two relatively equal proportions with one predominating
VPK	Doshas at almost equal proportions

V – Vata   P – Pitta   K – Kapha

find your Dosha

FIND OUT YOUR DOSHA TYPE (PRAKRITI OR BODY CONSTITUTION)

Check the choices that most closely match your tendencies throughout your life.

	VATA	PITTA	KAPHA	V	P	K
Body size	Thin	Medium	Large	☐	☐	☐
Weight	Light	Medium	Heavy	☐	☐	☐
Skin	Dry, cold, rough	Oily, flushed, warm	Soft, smooth, pale	☐	☐	☐
Complexion	Dark, dull	Red, glowing	Pale, white	☐	☐	☐
Hair	Dry, brittle, thin	Oily, gray, bald	Thick, full, lustrous	☐	☐	☐
Face	Oval	Triangular	Round	☐	☐	☐
Eyes	Small, dry, nervous	Medium, sharp, bright	Big, calm, loving	☐	☐	☐
Hands	Small, dry, cold	Medium, moist	Thick, firm	☐	☐	☐
Fingers	Thin, long	Medium, pointed	Large, stocky	☐	☐	☐
Joints	Small, cracking	Medium, moist	Large, lubricated	☐	☐	☐
Voice	Weak, hoarse	Strong tone	Deep, good tone	☐	☐	☐
Speech	Talkative, rapid	Clear, sharp	Quiet, slow	☐	☐	☐
Sleep	Irregular	Regular	Deep	☐	☐	☐
Activities	Hyperactive	Moderate	Sedentary	☐	☐	☐
Appetite	Irregular	Strong	Slow, steady	☐	☐	☐
Elimination	Constipated	Regular	Sluggish	☐	☐	☐
Emotions	Anxious, worried	Irritable, determined	Calm, attachment	☐	☐	☐
Memory	Variable	Selective	Detailed	☐	☐	☐
Mind	Restless	Impatient	Calm	☐	☐	☐
Hobbies	Art, dance, travel	Politics, sports	Reading, gardening	☐	☐	☐
Health	Anxiety, depression	Fevers, heartburn, skin	Congestion, allergies	☐	☐	☐
Weather	Warm, moist	Cool, temperate	Warm, dry	☐	☐	☐
			TOTAL			

dhatus

THE SEVEN TISSUES (SAPTA DHATU)

The human body is composed of seven basic dhatus, or tissues. These seven tissues are responsible for keeping the body structure together. They also play a very important role in nourishing the body. The grosser dhatus nourish the subtler dhatus, and the subtler dhatus protect the grosser dhatus.

They are:
Rasa, Rakta, Mamsa, Meda, Asthi, Majja, Shukra/Artava.

DHATU TISSUES	UPADATHU DERIVED FROM DHATUS	DHATU MALA BODY'S WASTE	FUNCTION
Rasa Plasma, lymph	Stanya (breast milk) Raja (menstruation)	Kapha (mucus)	Preenan (nourishment)
Rakta Blood	Sira (blood vessels) Kandara (tendons)	Pitta (bile)	Jeevana (giving life)
Mamsa Muscles and flesh	Vasa (subcutaneous fat) Twak (skin)	Khamala (waste from natural openings)	Lepana (plastering of body)
Meda Fat	Snayu (ligaments)	Sveda (sweat)	Snehana (lubrication)
Ashti Bone	Danta (teeth) Taruna (cartilage)	Kesha (hair) Nakha (nails)	Dharana (supporting the organs)
Majja Bone marrow	Ashru (tears)	Oily secretions in eyes, skin, feces	Poorana (filling, feeling)
Shukra/Artava Reproductive fluid	N/A	N/A	Reproduction

dhatus

CAUSES OF DHATUS DISORDERS

DHATUS	SIGNS AND SYMPTOMS OF DISORDERS
Rasa	**Rasa Vruddhi (increased)** – Frequent colds, sinus and bronchial congestion, swelling, water retention, excess salivation. **Rasa Kshaya (decreased)** – Dry skin, dehydration, dizziness, fatigue, excess thirst, palpitations.
Rakta	**Rakta Vruddhi (increased)** – Skin conditions (inflammation), enlarged liver or spleen. **Rakta Kshaya (decreased)** – Dry or rough skin, weakness, paralysis, numbness.
Mamsa	**Mamsa Vruddhi (increased)** – Enlarged glands, tumors, uterine fibroids. **Mamsa Kshaya (decreased)** – Atrophy and loss of muscle, emaciation, joint problems.
Meda	**Meda Vruddhi (increased)** – Obesity, sluggish metabolism, fatty tumors, diabetes. **Meda Kshaya (decreased)** – Weakness, cracking joints, bone loss, dilated spleen.
Ashti	**Ashti Vruddhi (increased)** – Spurs, bone tumors, calcification, extra teeth. **Ashti Kshaya (decreased)** – Rough or brittle nails, degenerative bone diseases, joint pain, fractures.
Majja	**Majja Vruddhi (increased)** – General heaviness, tumor on peripheral nerves. **Majja Kshaya (decreased)** – Bone loss, anemia, sciatica, dizziness.
Shukra/ Artava	**Shukra/Artava Vruddhi (increased)** – Increased sex, premature orgasm, ovarian cysts. **Shukra/Artava Kshaya (decreased)** – Low libido, low sperm count, impotence, sterility.

malas

WHAT IS MALA?
Mutra (urine), Purisha (feces), Sweda (sweat)

Malas are the body's waste products produced during the metabolic process. The effective elimination of malas from the body is crucial and vital for the maintenance of good health.

MALAS	
Mutra Urine	**Function** – removes water, salt and mineral wastes from the body. Helps maintain body fluid balanced and adequate blood pressure. **Imbalance** – bladder infection, fever, thirst, dehydration, frequent urination.
Purisha Feces	**Function** – removes toxins and solid wastes from the body; maintains tone and supports the intestinal wall. **Imbalance** – diarrhea or constipation, gas, hemorrhoids, parasites.
Sweda Sweat	**Function** – expels excess water and toxins. Keeps skin soft and maintains tone. Regulates the body temperature. **Imbalance** – dehydration, change in body temperature.

agni

AGNI, THE DIGESTIVE FIRE
The English word "ignite" originates from Sanskrit word "Agni" which simply means fire, responsible for digestion, metabolism, and conversion.

Agni converts food into body tissues. Agni represents all the heat processes responsible for maintaining body temperature, radiance, biochemical transformations, and electrical conduction. According to Ayurveda, life span, complexion, strength, health, enthusiasm, energy, vitality, and immune system depend on the state of one's agni. Agni mahabhuta represents the heating energy of Pitta.

We need to honor the digestive fire within us, which is primarily known as jathara agni. The conscious mind is intertwined with the mechanisms of the chemical process of digestion.

The following prayer will help with agni and digestion, if said before meals.

Annam Brahma raso Vishnu   The creative energy in the food is Brahma.
Pakto devo maheshvarah   The nourishing energy in the body is Vishnu.
Evam jñaktva tu yo bhunakte   The transformation of food into pure
Anna dosho na lipyate   consciousness is Shiva.

agni

MAIN TYPES OF AGNI

SUBDOSHA	
Jatharagni (1)	**Sites** Lower end of stomach and first part of duodenum. **Functions** It is the main fire that regulates all other agnis in the body. It is responsible for gross digestion.
Bhutagnis (5) Aakashiya Agni Vayaviya Agni Agniya Agni Aapya Agni Parthiv Agni	**Sites** Everywhere in the body and regulated by the liver. **Functions** It is responsible for the conversion of the five elements of ingested food into components that can be utilized by the body.
Dhatu Agni (7) Rasa Dhatu Agni Rakta Dhatu Agni Mamsa Dhatu Agni Meda Dhatu Agni Ashti Dhatu Agni Majja Dhatu Agni Shukra Dhatu Agni	**Sites** The membrane which functionally separates each dhatu. **Functions** Nourishment of all body tissues and transformation of immature into mature dhatu.

THE FOUR KINDS OF AGNI

STATE	EFFECT
Sama Agni (balanced)	**Related Dosha** – Tridoshic **Effect** – Digestion is regular, dhatus are balanced, and all body functions are normal. Perfect health.
Vishama Agni (irregular)	**Related Dosha** – Vata **Effect** – Variable digestion that will cause irregular appetite. Variable dhatu state.
Teekshna Agni (sharp)	**Related Dosha** – Pitta **Effect** – Fast digestion, desire to have large meals, or eat frequently. Most Pitta disorders are caused by this kind of agni.
Manda Agni (slow or weak)	**Related Dosha** – Kapha **Effect** – Food is not digested properly due to weak agni. The dhatus that are formed are of poor quality.

Ama

WHAT IS AMA?
Undigested food

Ama is created during the digestive process whereby incomplete or partially digested food matter is left behind in the digestive system. If not eliminated, this ama can turn harmful, affecting doshas and dhatus.

Ama is a unique concept in Ayurveda and it is linked to digestion. When ama gets mixed with doshas or malas, it is called "Sama" ("Sa" means with) and when it gets detached, it is called "Nirama" ("Nir" means without).

SYMPTOMS OF AMA

You wake up tired and don't feel fresh after a good night sleep.

You feel heavy, lethargic, sleepy and experience a lack of energy.

Your tongue is coated with white, sticky mucus when you wake up in the morning.

You don't feel real hunger and taste.

You feel generalized aches and pains, stiffness in the body.

You lack mental clarity or concentration.

You feel a sense of heaviness in the abdomen or in the body as a whole.

You experience frequent indigestion, gas, bloating, and stomach aches.

You experience stagnation in the body, like constipation, sinus congestion, and difficulty breathing.

HOW TO REDUCE AND TREAT AMA

Follow appropriate dietary rules according to your dosha to avoid formation of ama.

If ama has formed already, dietary regulations, herbal preparations, and fasting are recommended to digest ama.

When ama is already absorbed in the tissues, panchakarma treatments are recommended.

OPPOSITE QUALITIES OF AMA AND AGNI

AMA	AGNI		AMA	AGNI
Cold	Hot		Moist	Dry
Heavy	Light		Foul	Aromatic
Slimy	Rough		Stable	Mobile

srotas

WHAT ARE SROTAS?

Srotas are the major transportation system in the body. The literal meaning of the word sru means to flow.

The body channels carry solids, liquids, gases, nerve impulses, nutrients, waste products, and secretions in and out of the human physiology.

The human body is a network of appropriate nutrients and energies flowing through the channels, resulting in a healthy body and mind. Any kind of blockage, deficiency, or excess in the channels can result in various diseases.

In order to keep srotas healthy, regular yogic exercises, pranayama, cleansing, and daily hygienic regimens are recommended.

The human body possesses two main circulation channels (srotas), although Ayurveda recognizes 11 other such channels.

One circulation channel digests consumed nutrients, that are transported from the gastrointestinal tract into the cells and tissues. This nourishes the body.

This channel also carries the right proportions of the doshas (constituted of the mahabhutas) and the other basic tissue elements from one part of the body to another. This mechanism keeps the body healthy.

The other pathway transports waste products produced by the body, to be eliminated naturally via the malas.

The body channels are classified in two categories: internal channels and external channels.

There are thirteen srotas in the internal channels. Three srotas connect the individual to the external environment by inhaling and exhaling air, and ingesting food and water. Seven srotas are associated with the seven dhatus or tissues. The other three srotas eliminate the metabolic waste from the body.

srotas

THE THREE SROTAS THAT CONNECT THE INDIVIDUAL TO THE EXTERNAL ENVIRONMENT

SROTAS	FUNCTION
Prana vaha	Carries the breath to all parts of the body
Anna vaha	Transports solid and liquid foods
Udaka vaha	Transports water

THE SEVEN SROTAS ASSOCIATED WITH THE SEVEN DHATUS OR TISSUES

SROTAS	FUNCTION
Rasa vaha	Carries plasma and lymph
Rakta vaha	Carries blood cells, specially hemoglobin
Mamsa vaha	Carries muscle nutrients and wastes
Meda vaha	Supplies adipose tissues
Asthi vaha	Carries nutrients to bones and transports wastes
Majja vaha	Supplies bone marrow and nerves, including the brain
Shukra vaha	Carries the sperm and ova and supplies nutrients to them

THE THREE SROTAS ASSOCIATED WITH ELIMINATION OF METABOLIC WASTE FROM THE BODY

SROTAS	FUNCTION
Purisha vaha	Carries feces
Mutra vaha	Carries urine
Sweda vaha	Carries sweat

digestion according to Ayurveda

GROSS DIGESTION
The Three Stages of Digestion

Usually it takes from four to six hours to digest a meal. The length of time may depend on the quality of agni and the individual constitution. Each stage relates to a different taste.

THREE STAGES	
First Stage	**Madhura Avastha Paka (sweet)** Dominant dosha – Kapha Location – mouth and stomach Elements extracted – water and earth Excess – causes mucus, profuse salivation, poor appetite
Second Stage	**Amla Avastha Paka (sour)** Dominant dosha – Pitta Location – stomach and small intestine Elements extracted – fire Excess – causes ulcers, hyperacidity
Third Stage	**Katu Avastha Paka (pungent)** Dominant dosha – Vata Location – large intestine Elements extracted – air and ether Excess – causes gas, constipation

SUBTLE DIGESTION
The Three Laws of Nutrition

The three laws of nutrition are Kedari Kulya Nyaya (Irrigation), Khale Kapot Nyaya (Selectivity), Ksheer Dadhi Nyaya (Transformation). These processes happen at a subtle level after gross digestion is completed. At this point, dhatu nourishment is initialized. At each level of dhatu digestion four products are formed: Asthayi Dhatu, Sthayi Dhatu, Upadhatu, Dhatu Mala.

LAW 1 – KEDARI KULYA NYAYA

Law of irrigation – circulation of nutrients to dhatus.

LAW 2 – KHALE KAPOT NYAYA

Law of selectivity – each dhatu selects appropriate nutrients.

LAW 3 – KSHEER DADHI NYAYA

Law of transformation – conversion of Ashtaya Dhatu (unprocessed) into Sthayi Dhatu (stable mature).

secret of your health

OJAS

According to the principles of Ayurveda, it is the essential energy of the body which can be equated with the "fluid of life".

The concept of ojas in Ayurveda is very subtle and remarkable. Ojas is produced at every stage of digestion and is the finest end product. As such, it is the essence of all body tissues (dhatus).

According to Sushruta, "ojas is the sap of one's life energy". Sufficient ojas generates vigor, strength, zest for life, and a strong immune system. Deficient ojas causes debility, weariness, and eventually disease. It contains prana and it is the link between material and spiritual.

One of many ojas functions are to maintain quantity and quality of dhatus, malas, and doshas. It supports the body and it is a source of natural strength to fight off diseases. It enables the body-mind's balanced functioning. Ojas is responsible for sustaining immunity, health, and strength. Following a sattvic life style and diet will increase ojas. Overexertion, excessive anger, grief, thinking, worry, anxiety, and injury/harm to the body decreases ojas.

There are two types of ojas: para and apara. Para ojas is superior and Apara ojas is inferior.

PARA OJAS

Which is eight drops in quantity and located in the heart, extremely vital, and its loss leads to immediate death.

APARA OJAS

Which is half an anjali (amounting to cupping both palms together), is all over your body and circulates through ten major blood vessels (dasha maha mula dhamanis) to the entire body.

OPPOSITE QUALITIES OF ALCOHOL AND OJAS

OJAS	ALCOHOL		OJAS	ALCOHOL
Sweet	Sour		Heavy	Light
Cold	Hot		Dull	Sharp
Oily	Dry		Gross	Subtle
Stable	Mobile		Slimy	Clear
Smooth	Rough		Clear	Spreading

nutrition and Diet

AYURVEDA WISDOM AND NUTRITION

Ayurveda mentions that "a person who eats a wholesome diet, does not require medicine, and no medicine will cure a person who does not eat a wholesome diet".

The science of nutrition has developed over time, but Ayurveda has a different view regarding diet.

There is a simple distinction between modern dietetics and Ayurvedic diet. Modern dietetics classifies food by groups such as carbohydrates, fats, proteins, minerals and vitamins, and focus on calorie intake.

Ayurveda gives more importance to the nature of food, preparation, tastes, quantity and quality. It also takes into consideration the individual constitution, the digestive capacity intake, and food combinations.

The six Tastes

THE SIX TASTES (RASA)
Ra-taste, relish or praise | sa-juice, sap or secretion

Taste is perceived through the tongue (sense organ) and it has a great impact in our senses through the intake of food.

There are six tastes consisting of two combinations of the five elements (bhoutic composition). The six tastes also have a cooling or heating energy that will increase or decrease the doshas.

TASTE	ELEMENTS	ENERGY	VATA	PITTA	KAPHA
Madhura I Sweet	Earth + Water	Cold	↓	↓	↑
Amla I Sour	Earth + Fire	Hot	↓	↑	↑
Lavana I Salty	Water + Fire	Hot	↓	↑	↑
Katu I Pungent	Fire + Air	Hot	↑	↑	↓
Tikta I Bitter	Air + Ether	Cold	↑	↓	↓
Kashaya I Astringent	Air + Earth	Cold	↑	↓	↓

the six tastes

TASTES AND THE BODY

MADHURA | SWEET

Promotes growth and strengthens all body tissues, contributes to healthy skin and hair.
Some examples: complex carbohydrates, grains, root vegetables (potatoes, beets), sugar, honey, maple syrup, milk, dates.

AMLA | SOUR

Energizes the body, increases salivary secretion, stimulates appetite, enhances attention.
Some examples: sour cream, yogurt, sour fruits, vinegar, cheese, fermented foods.

LAVANA | SALTY

Strengthens agni, aids digestion, maintains water electrolyte balance, helps eliminate waste.
Some examples: salts – rock, sea, gypsum and black; seaweed and tamari.

KATU | PUNGENT

Improves digestion and absorption, reduces congestion, anticoagulant, aids circulation, antispasmodic, anti-parasitic.
Some examples: black pepper, cayenne pepper, chili pepper, pippali, onion, garlic, ginger, radish.

TIKTA | BITTER

Eliminates toxins, anti-inflammatory, antipyretic, laxative, liver and digestive tonic.
Some examples: leafy vegetables, neen, golden seal, aloe vera, fenugreek, black tea, myrrh, bitter melon, coffee, sandalwood.

KASHAYA | ASTRINGENT

Improves absorption, constricts blood vessels, stops bleeding, promotes healing, antidiuretic, anti-bacterial, homeostatic.
Some examples: chickpeas, green beans, alum, unripe banana, turmeric, golden seal, blueberries, cranberries, beans.

TASTES AND THE MIND

TASTE	EFFECT ON THE MIND	IN EXCESS
Madhura	Sweet	Compassion, love	Attachment, heaviness
Amla	Sour	Perception, stimulation	Discontent, jealousy, anger
Lavana	Salty	Conviction, passion for life	Greed, overly ambitious
Katu	Pungent	Focused, sharp, attentive	Cruelty, hostility, envy
Tikta	Bitter	Satisfaction, self awareness	Grief, depletion
Kashaya	Astringent	Quiet	Anxiety, fear

diet quality

SATTVIC, RAJASIC AND TAMASIC DIET

According to its features, foods you eat are either sattvic, rajasic, or tamasic and exert different effects upon the body and mind.

Sattva is the quality of purity and light; rajas is the quality of movement and change; tamas is the quality of inertia and darkness.

Food and diet can be categorized into three groups:

Sattvic food is the purest form of food. It promotes clarity and feelings of contentment. It is easily digested, brings harmony to the mind, and nourishes the body. It is the best food for yoga practitioners. Sattvic food includes ghee, honey, herbs, nuts, seeds, legumes, cow's milk, fresh fruits, vegetables, beans, and whole grains.

Rajasic food is stimulating and in excess creates mind-body imbalance. It tends to over-stimulate the body and makes the mind restless. In moderation, helps to kindle agni and activates vital energy. This food is spicy, salty, dry, sour, hot, and bitter.

Spicy food is tempting, stimulating to the senses, and agitating to the mind.

Rajasic food includes salt, eggs, white sugar, tea, coffee, vinegar, and hot spices.

Tamasic food is lifeless. It clouds reasoning, creates lethargy, depletes the body of energy, and debilitates the immune system. It also invokes feelings of anger, jealousy, and greed in people. Overeating is a tamasic behavior.

Tamasic food includes meat, alcohol, tobacco, onions, garlic, as well fermented, stale, deep fried, and frozen foods.

Tamasic foods should be avoided.

AYURVEDIC DIET AND SEASON

Changing seasons cause change in the levels of the doshas (body constitution). To maintain balance, one must adapt the diet accordingly.

Sweet, bitter, and astringent foods should be eaten more frequently in the fall. In early winter eat more sweet, sour, and salty foods. In late winter eat more pungent, bitter, and astringent foods. In Spring eat more astringent, bitter, and pungent tastes. In summer eat more sweet, bitter, and astringent foods. In the rainy season eat more sour, salty, and sweet foods.

Foods have generally a heating or cooling quality. Depending on the body-type, the season, and the weather adjust eating habits on a daily basis. For example, in summer, if it is a cold day, eat more heating foods on that day. If feeling hot on any given day, eat more cooling foods.

Diet according to your Dosha

VATA DOSHA DIET

Vata predominant constitution should select a diet which is calming, soothing and nourishing.

Vata's food should be warm, moist and heavy. Sweet, sour, and salty tastes are favored over pungent, bitter, and astringent tastes. Meals should be small and frequent, but regular. Warm, steamed, or cooked foods are settling. Raw food, fast food, dried food, and frozen foods should be avoided.

VATA	PACIFYING DIET
Fruits	Apricots, avocados, bananas, berries, coconut, dates, figs, grapes, mangoes, melons, nectarines, passion fruit, oranges, peaches, plums, prunes.
Vegetables	Asparagus, beets, carrots, cucumber, eggplant, leek, lentils (red), mung beans (green gram), mustard greens, pumpkin, radish, squash, sweet potatoes.
Spices	Anise, cayenne, cinnamon, cumin, garlic, ginger, mustard, thyme.
Grains	Basmati rice, couscous, oats (cooked), quinoa, spelt, wheat.
Nuts & Seeds	Almonds, cashews, pumpkin seed, pistachios, sesame seeds, sunflower seeds, walnuts.
Dairy	Buttermilk, cheeses, cottage cheese, cow's milk (unhomogenized), ghee, kefir, yogurt.
Meats	Beef, chicken, eggs, fish, turkey.
Supplements	Dietary fiber, probiotic.
MEALS	SAMPLE
Breakfast	Spiced oatmeal with fruit. Cream of wheat. Wheat bread with ghee. Herbal teas, fennel and cardamom tea.
Lunch	Vegetable stews, rice, bread.
Dinner	Steamed vegetables, soups, rice.

Diet according to your Dosha

PITTA DOSHA DIET

Pitta predominant constitution should select a diet which is cooling and moderately heavy.

Pitta's food should be cool or warm, and moderately heavy. Sweet, bitter, and astringent tastes are favored over sour, salty, and pungent tastes. Meals should be regular. Food is better warm, steamed, or cooked. Processed, fermented, spicy, fast foods, and alcoholic beverages should be avoided.

PITTA	PACIFYING DIET
Fruits	Apples, avocados, figs, grapes, mangoes, melons, oranges, pears, pineapples, plums, prunes, raisins.
Vegetables	Asparagus, broccoli, cabbage, cauliflower, celery, leafy green vegetables, mushrooms, peas, potatoes, sprouts, sweet potatoes, zucchini.
Spices & Herbs	Cardamom, cilantro, cinnamon, coriander, dill, fennel, mint, saffron, turmeric.
Grains	Basmati rice, barley, couscous, oats, wheat.
Nuts & Seeds	Pumpkin seeds, sunflower seeds.
Dairy	Butter, ghee, ice cream, milk, yogurt.
Meats	Chicken, shrimp, turkey.
Supplements	Aloe vera, wheat grass.
MEALS	SAMPLE
Breakfast	Fresh fruit salad, wheat toast. Mint tea.
Lunch	Salads, vegetables, pasta, meat sandwich.
Dinner	Vegetables, soups, rice.

diet according to your dosha

KAPHA DOSHA DIET

Kapha predominant constitution should select a diet which is warming and stimulating.

Kapha's food should be warm and light. Pungent, bitter and astringent tastes are favored over sweet, sour, salty tastes. Small and light meals are preferable. Food is better if it is lightly cooked. Raw fruits, vegetables and salads are recommended. Spicy food is good for Kapha to stimulate digestion. Avoid processed, fried, and fast foods.

KAPHA	PACIFYING DIET
Fruits	Apples, apricots, cranberries, pears, pomegranates.
Vegetables	Asparagus, beets, broccoli, cabbage, carrots, celery, garlic, leafy green vegetables, lettuce, mushrooms, onions, spinach, sprouts, turnip, watercress.
Spices & Herbs	Black pepper, chili pepper, horseradish, mustard, scallions, sprouts.
Grains	Barley, buckwheat, corn, couscous, millet, muesli, oats (dry), quinoa, rye.
Nuts & Seeds	Flax, pumpkin and sunflower seeds.
Dairy	Low and non-fat milk.
Meats	Chicken, fish, shrimp, turkey, venison.
Supplements	Bitter greens.
MEALS	SAMPLE
Breakfast	Fresh fruit salad. Toast with light butter. Quinoa cereal.
Lunch	Vegetable, sandwich with light meat, salads.
Dinner	Pasta with vegetables, rice, soups.

spices

THE IMPORTANCE OF SPICES

According to Ayurveda, food plays an important role in prevention. Proper intake of nutritious food according to body constitution is necessary for good health. Also the right combination of foods and the amount ingested play an important role in preserving health. Ayurveda also advises that most diseases occur from improper eating habits and poor nutrition. By using spices at every meal, your agni (digestive fire) and digestion are enhanced, therefore leading to health and well-being. Spices also have a therapeutic effect.

The "spice-box" or seven spices are considered the magic of Indian cooking. The exotic colors and aromas can stimulate your olfactory sensory organ and taste buds that aids in digestion and balance your mind and body.

GENERAL TIPS FOR COOKING WITH SPICES

Most spices are potent, so you need only a little amount.

These seven combinations of spices are suitable for each body type, but you can blend them as per your taste. These are combinations of sattvic, rajasic and tamasic spices.

SPICES	TASTE	QUALITY	DHATU AFFECTED
Cumin seeds	Bitter	Heating	Plasma I Rasa
Turmeric	Bitter, pungent, astringent	Heating	Blood I Rakta
Mustard seeds	Pungent	Heating	Muscles I Meda
Coriander	Bitter, pungent	Cooling	Fat I Mansa
Fenugreek seeds	Bitter, astringent	Heating	Bones I Ashti
Asafoetida	Pungent	Heating	Nerves I Majja
Ginger powder	Pungent, bitter, sweet	Heating	Reproductive I Shukra

spices

SEVEN IMPORTANT SPICES

C U M I N (Cuminum cyminum) | Related dhatu – rasa

Action – diuretic, carminative, stimulant, astringent, antispasmodic.

Uses – valuable in dyspepsia, diarrhea, hoarseness, flatulence and colic.

Effect on dosha – V ↑ P ↑ K ↓   **Energetics** – pungent/hot/pungent

C O R I A N D E R (Coriandrum sativum) | Related dhatu – mamsa

Action – carminative, digestive stimulating, tonic.

Uses – headache and swelling; essential oil in colic, rheumatism and neuralgia; the seeds as a paste for mouth ulceration and a poultice for other ulcers.

Effect on dosha – V ↓ P ↓ K ↓   **Energetics** – bitter/pungent-cold-pungent

T U R M E R I C (Curcuma domestica) | Related dhatu – rakta

Action – mild digestive, aromatic, stimulant, carminative.

Uses – anemia, blood purifier, circulation, indigestion, skin disorders, all inflammatory conditions.

Effect on dosha – V ↑ P ↑ K ↓   **Energetics** – bitter/astringent/pungent-hot-pungent

M U S T A R D (Brassica alba) | Related dhatu – meda

Action – stimulant, demulcent, emetic (induce vomiting).

Uses – epilepsy, toothache, bruises, stiff neck, rheumatism, colic, and respiratory troubles.

Effect on dosha – V ↓ P ↓ K ↑   **Energetics** – pungent/hot/pungent

A S A F O E T I D A / H I N G (Ferula assafoetida) | Related dhatu – majja

Action – digestive, analgesic, stimulant, carminative, antispasmodic.

Uses – flatulence, respiratory conditions like asthma, bronchitis, whooping cough.

Effect on dosha – V ↓ P ↑ K ↓   **Energetics** – pungent/heating/pungent

spices

SEVEN IMPORTANT SPICES

FENUGREEK (Trigonella foenum-graecum) | Related dhatu – ashti

Action – diuretic, tonic, stimulant.

Uses – digestive aid, boils, cysts, lowers blood pressure.

Effect on dosha – V ↑ P ↑ K ↓   **Energetics** – pungent/hot/pungent

GINGER (Zingiber officinale) | Related dhatu – shukra

Action – aphrodisiac, carminative, diaphoretic, digestive, expectorant, stimulant.

Uses – colic, vomiting, indigestion, flatulence, colds, cough, asthma, congestive conditions.

Effect on dosha – V ↓ P ↑ K ↓   **Energetics** – pungent/sweet-hot-sweet

SATTVIC, RAJASIC AND TAMASIC SPICES

SATTVIC SPICES	RAJASIC SPICES	TAMASIC SPICES
Cardamom	Black pepper	Red pepper
Saffron	Cumin	Mustard
Cinnamon	Hing	Garlic

Light Diet

AYURVEDIC APPROACH TO A LIGHT DIET

According to Ayurveda, it is important to know how and what to eat when your agni (digestive fire) is low. It might be during or while recuperating from an illness, or during panchakarma.

During these periods your digestive system becomes weak and functions below its optimal levels. Agni becomes weak and one has to gradually increase the strength of the digestive fire to regain energy and health.

When the digestive fire is low, if you consume heavy foods, ama will accumulate in the digestive system. A light diet gives more time and energy for your digestive system to digest ama.

Ayurveda suggests rice and mung beans/lentils as a light diet, because they cook and digest easily. They also balance all three doshas.

One of the famous recipes named khichadi, a nutritious combination of rice, mung beans, vegetables, spices, seeds and ghee, is an excellent one-dish meal for people on lighter diets.

Kanji water is a special warm drink made from either split mung beans or organic brown rice.

One to two quarts of warm kanji water can be drunk throughout the day, between light meals. Kanji water provides instant nutrition to the cell walls, because of the lightness of rice and beans. It provides carbohydrates, giving the body energy and strength. It also provides sustenance during illnesses like diarrhea, fever, and dehydration.

LIGHT DIET SAMPLE	
Breakfast	Stewed apples and pears, or hot cereal.
Lunch	Soupy split mung dahl, basmati rice or quinoa, vegetables sauteed in ghee and spices.
Dinner	Khichadi, vegetable soup, or steamed veggies.
Foods	**Favor** Mung dahl, aduki beans, basmati rice, barley, quinoa, tofu, cooked vegetables with ghee. Spices such as turmeric, cumin, ginger, fennel, black pepper and coriander. Hot milk with ginger, stewed fruit, fruit and fresh vegetable juices, ripe sweet fruit, sunflower and sesame seeds, lassi, dates, figs, raisins, ghee and olive oil. **Avoid** Hard cheeses, eggs, fish, meat, chicken. If meat is on your diet then Ayurveda recommends having it during the day time in the form of a soup that has cooked for a long time.

Recipes

KHICHADI OR MUNG BEAN AND BASMATI RICE STEW

Khichadi is the easiest solid food to digest.

Ayurveda offers khichadi, a recipe that can heal various diseases. This recipe is used in Ayurvedic cleansing therapy, because of its ease of digestion and assimilation. This is especially good during the transition of the seasons.

This is also known as sattvic food, suitable for anyone at any age. The great thing about khichadi is that additional spices or vegetables can be added to this recipe according to one's constitution.

Split mung beans (or dahl) can be found at most health food stores.

Basmati rice is the most digestible. Be sure to add even more water, as the rice absorbs it quickly, and khichadi should be thin and runny.

Ingredients
½ cup basmati rice
¼ cup split mung beans
3-4 cups water
2-3 teaspoon ghee or olive oil
¼ teaspoon mustard seeds, ¼ teaspoon fenugreek seeds
½ teaspoon cumin seeds
1 pinch of red chili or cayenne pepper
1 teaspoon freshly grated ginger
¼ teaspoon asafoetida powder (also known as hing)
¼ teaspoon turmeric, salt to taste like 1/8 to 1/4 teaspoon
2 cups chopped vegetables like zucchini, carrots, leeks
4-5 stems cilantro, washed and chopped
½ cup spinach leaves, washed and finely chopped
1-2 teaspoon dry shredded coconut
1 teaspoon lemon juice

Preparation
Sort through the mung beans and remove any debris, such as rocks or sticks.

Rinse the mung beans and rice in a fine mesh strainer and set aside.

In a pot, heat the ghee or oil on medium heat and add mustard seeds, fenugreek seeds, cumin seeds, hing, turmeric, red chili, and ginger in this order and saute for 1-2 minutes. Add the mung beans, basmati rice, and vegetables then add water and salt. Bring to a boil and then turn the heat to low. Cook for about 30 to 40 minutes or until mung beans are soft and completely cooked. Top with cilantro leaves, coconut, and spinach, add fresh lemon juice at the end, and stir nicely.

Preparation Time: 45 minutes

Recipes

KANJI

Ingredients

7 parts water
1 part organic brown rice, a pinch of salt, fresh ground ginger, cumin

Preparation

Bring water and rice to a boil. Allow to boil until the rice becomes swollen and broken. Stir and strain out rice. However, it is not necessary to strain out small pieces of rice. Add a pinch each of ginger, ground cumin and salt. Pour into a thermos and drink throughout the day.

LENTIL SOUP

Ingredients

½ cup of french lentils or mung beans
½ pinch asafoetida
½ teaspoon turmeric powder
4-5 stems of cilantro — washed and chopped
1/8 teaspoon chili powder
2- 3 teaspoon olive oil or ghee
½ cup washed, chopped greens like spinach, kale
1 teaspoon coriander seed powder
¼ teaspoon mustard seeds
½ teaspoon cumin seeds
Salt to taste

Preparation

Wash the dhal in 2-3 changes of water, until the water is clear.

Drain. Add 2 cups of water to dhal and allow it to boil for 6-10 minutes, until dhal is soft. Whisk it with a spoon until smooth. Add greens, like spinach or kale. Simmer for 10-15 minutes. Heat the oil in a fry pan and sauté mustard seeds; when it breaks, add cumin seeds, turmeric, asafoetida, coriander powder and chili powder. Add this spicy oil into the dhal and mix properly. Finish with cilantro leaves and salt to taste. Serve with rice.

Preparation Time: 30 minutes

Recipes

AYURVEDIC VEGETABLE SOUP

The unique blend of herbs and vegetables makes this soup balance all three doshas.

Ingredients

1 big onion
½ cabbage
1 medium carrot
1 small yam
1 tablespoon olive oil
5 cups water
1 ½ teaspoons grated ginger
1 ½ teaspoon coriander powder
¼ teaspoon cayenne
½ teaspoon cumin powder
½ teaspoon turmeric powder
1 teaspoon salt
1 tablespoon lemon juice

Preparation

Wash all the vegetables and chop finely.
Heat oil in a big pot. Add onion and sauté for 3 minutes. Add the other vegetables and sauté for 2 minutes. Add 2 cups of water, ginger, turmeric, cayenne, and salt and cook for 10 minutes. Add coriander and cumin powder and cook for 15 more minutes. Add 3 cups of water and cook for 5 more minutes. Before serving, add lemon juice and mix well.

Serve hot.

Preparation Time: 30 minutes

Recipes

GHEE

In Ayurveda, ghee is a sacred and celebrated symbol of auspiciousness and plays an important role because of its healing properties.

Ghee is sweet in taste and has a cooling potency. It is anti-aging, nourishing, rejuvenating, good for the eyes, kindles agni, improves digestion, enhances memory, intellect, stamina, immune system, and promotes longevity.

Ghee is made by cooking butter to remove all milk solids and water; what is left is a pure golden oil with a royal flavor and aroma. Ghee can be used for cooking, sautéing, stir-frying, deep-frying, baking, flavoring popcorn, or used as a spread.

Ingredients

1 pound unsalted organic butter
Cheesecloth or muslin cloth or fine strainer
Heavy-bottomed cook pot
1 clean glass jar with lid

Preparation

Melt the butter over medium heat gradually in a heavy-bottomed pot. Do not stir.

Cook the melted butter until it is a clear golden liquid. It may bubble some, and foam may form on top, but do not skim off the foam. Golden or light brown solids will form and may settle at the bottom.

Butter usually begins to boil with lots of bubbles. When it is done, it will have foam on top of it, indicating that ghee is nearly done.

Remove from heat while the liquid is a clear gold.
A darker color means overdone ghee.

When it is warm, carefully strain the ghee through the cheesecloth or with a fine strainer into a clean, dry glass jar. Close with a lid when it becomes cold.

Note

Ghee at room temperature looks semi-solid.

Ghee does not need to be refrigerated.

Always use a clean utensil to scoop out ghee.

Preparation Time: 30 minutes

prevention

WHAT IS SWASTHA VRITTA?
Swa-self | stha-established | vritta-science or information

Prevention is a very important characteristic in Ayurveda and it enforces the great significance of being attuned into the rhythms of nature.

In order to achieve good health, prevent diseases, and attain the four goals of life, it is critical that one is in harmony with nature. Observing the changes of seasons, daily and nightly cycles, birth and aging patterns, and adjusting one's life style to these cycles, ensure a successful and healthy life.

THE DOSHAS AND THE LIFE CYCLES

VATA	PITTA	KAPHA
Dominant	Dominant	Dominant
during old age	in mid life	in childhood
50 – death	20 – 50 years of age	birth – 20 years of age

Pitta
PUBERTY   MIDDLE
Vata
BIRTH | DEATH
Kapha

THE FOUR PURUSHARTHAS OR GOALS OF LIFE
Purusha means an individual or person, and Artha means objective, pursuit or meaning.

According to the Vedic System, there are four major goals or objectives in life.

The four Purusharthas are Kama, Artha, Dharma and Moksha.

KAMA | DESIRE

The fulfillment of one's desires.

ARTHA | WEALTH

The pursuit of material wealth.

DHARMA | RIGHTEOUSNESS, DUTY

The duties and work one needs to do during different stages of life.

MOKSHA | LIBERATION

The ultimate goal in life. It is the experience of realizing the self and being one with the Universe.

prevention

DAILY ROUTINES | DINACHARYA

WAKING UP	
Time	Sattva time 5 – 6 am

CLEANSING	
Teeth	Should be cleaned morning, night, and after meals. Use a soft toothbrush and a mixture of astringent, pungent, and bitter herbs. There are commercial toothpastes and powders available at natural food stores.
Tongue (Scraping)	Scrape every morning and any other time that the teeth are brushed. Use a stainless steel scraper made of gold, silver, or copper. **Benefits** Cleanses coated tongue, removes bacteria, and stimulates gastric fire.
Gargling	Triphala decoction. **Benefits** Strengthens teeth, gums, and improves oral hygiene.
Face	VATA – warm water PITTA – cool water KAPHA – warm water **Benefits** Removes sweat, and natural secretions; improves circulation, prevents skin infections, acne, and discoloration of the skin.
Eyes	Wash with water at room temperature. Rotate eyes in clockwise direction and then in counter-clockwise direction; up and down; side to side. **Benefits** Prevents eye problems, enhances vision, reduces discharges.
Whole Body	Bathe at least once a day, as it is refreshing and cleansing. **Benefits** Cleanses the skin of sweat and impurities. Brings alertness and energy to the body and reduces fatigue.

EXERCISE	
Physical Exercise	Everyday exercise is beneficial to everyone. The exercise you choose will depend on your constitutional type (prakriti). Yoga stretches are recommended for all constitutions. **Benefits** Reduces fat, fatigue and lethargy. Builds and tones muscles, increases endurance, improves digestion.

prevention

DAILY ROUTINES | DINACHARYA

MASSAGE			
Whole Body	Gently massage head and body with warm oil.		
	VATA – Sesame oil	PITTA – Coconut oil	KAPHA – Sesame oil
	Benefits Prevents aging, improves circulation, reduces Vata dosha, calms the mind. Soften the skin, prevents wrinkles.		

PERFUMES	VATA	PITTA	KAPHA
Aromatherapy	Aromas should be calming and pacifying	Aromas should be cooling and sweet	Aromas should be stimulating and spicy
	Basil, orange, geranium, clove, and rose	Sandalwood, mint, rose, and jasmine	Juniper, ginger, eucalyptus, clove, and saffron

MEALTIME	VATA	PITTA	KAPHA
Breakfast	Moderate	Heavy	Light or skip
Lunch	11 am – noon	noon	noon – 1 pm
Supper	6 – 7 pm	6 – 7 pm	6 – 7 pm
After meals	Take a 15-20 minutes nap lying on your left side, or take a leisurely walk.		

NIGHTLY ROUTINES | RITUCHARYA

BEDTIME	
Sleep	Things that promote sleep: Oil massaged on the soles of feet and scalp A cup of hot milk Meditation
Sex	Spring and fall sex should be reduced to twice a week. Summer once a week. Winter sex can be performed daily or alternate days.

prevention

SEASONAL ROUTINES | RITUCHARYA

FALL & WINTER	VATA SEASON
Diet	Foods and drinks with warm, moist, and heavy qualities to counter the dry, cold, and light qualities of Vata. **Food** Oatmeal, cream of wheat, tapioca. Stews, soups and gravies, steamed vegetables, basmati rice, mung dal khichadi. Nuts such as pecans and almonds. **Avoid** Salads, raw vegetables. Pungent, astringent, and bitter tastes. **Favor** Sweet, salty, and sour tastes.
Drinks	Herbal teas made with cumin-coriander-fennel, or ginger-cinnamon. A cup of warm milk at bedtime. Avoid cold drinks.
Massage	Apply warm sesame oil throughout the body and take a warm shower.
Exercise	**Yoga** Alternate nostril pranayama. Poses such as lotus, forward and backward bends, vajrasana, spinal twist, camel, cobra and cat asanas. Sun salutations, in moderation.
Sleep	Take a short afternoon nap.
Dress	Wear warm colors such as red, yellow, and orange.
Herbs	Dashmul, ashvaghanda, bala, vidari, and brahmi.

prevention

SEASONAL ROUTINES | RITUCHARYA

SPRING	KAPHA SEASON
Diet	Food and drinks with hot, dry, light qualities to counter the cool, moist, and heavy qualities of Kapha. **Food** Baked, broiled, or grilled warm foods. Legumes, vegetables, and hot spices. **Avoid** Sweet, salty, and sour foods. Dairy products. Heavy, oily foods and cold drinks. **Add** Pungent, bitter, and astringent foods.
Drinks	Should be made with ginger, calamus and clove. Emphasize herbal teas (cumin, coriander and fennel). Warm water.
Massage	Use dry herbal powders such as haritaki, ginger, or heating oil.
Exercise	**Yoga** Bhastrika pranayama. Poses such as sun salutations, fish, boat, bow, lion and camel poses, head stand or shoulder stand.
Sleep	**Avoid** Sleeping during the day.
Dress	Bright warm colors like gold, orange.
Herbs	Pippali, black pepper, ginger, and purnanava.

prevention

SEASONAL ROUTINES | RITUCHARYA

SUMMER	PITTA SEASON
Diet	Cool, heavy, bland foods and drinks to counter the hot, bright, and sharp qualities of Pitta. **Food** Salads, basmati rice, steamed vegetables, cucumber raita. Light meat, turkey or chicken. Melons, plums, pears, and apples. **Avoid** Hot, spicy, sour, and pungent tastes and hot drinks. **Add** Fruit and more vegetables.
Drinks	Lassi, lime juice, and coconut water.
Massage	In the morning with coconut or sunflower oil.
Exercise	Swimming, walking on green grass. **Yoga** Shitali Pranayama. Poses such as cow, cobra, fish, boat, palm tree asanas. Moon salutation.
Sleep	Take a short nap after lunch.
Dress	Cotton or silk clothing. Colors such as white, grey, purple, green.
Herbs	Amalaki, sandalwood, shatavari, guduchi, licorice, pomegranate.

Doshas General Guidelines

BALANCING VATA

The key to balancing Vata is regularity.

Regular habits, quietness, and attention to fluids.

Decrease stress.

Emphasize ample rest, warmth and a steady supply of nourishment.

Stay warm – being a cold dosha, Vata benefits from heat.

Eat a Vata pacifying diet, and eat regularly.

Drink lots of warm fluids during the day to prevent dehydration.

Avoid mental strain and over-stimulation.

Do not drink alcohol while you are trying to balance Vata, which resents stimulants of any kind, including coffee, tea, and nicotine.

BALANCING PITTA

The key to balancing Pitta is moderation.

Moderation, coolness, and attention to leisure.

Emphasize balance of rest and activity.

Coolness in any form helps to counteract overactive Pitta.

Eat a Pitta pacifying diet. It's important not to overeat.

Avoid artificial stimulants, all of which raise Pitta.

Avoid strenuous physical exertion or overheating yourself outdoors.

Make sure to go outdoors as much as possible.

BALANCING KAPHA

The key to balancing Kapha is stimulation.

Stimulation, regular exercise, and weight control.

Emphasize variety in life.

Eat a Kapha pacifying diet – it is important not to overeat if you are a Kapha type.

Reduce sweets.

Stay warm. Kapha benefits from heat.

Avoid damp.

Drink warm fluids during the day, but in moderation.

Exercise regularly, preferably every day.

panchakarma

WHAT IS PANCHAKARMA

Panchakarma is a Sanskrit word that means "five actions" or "five treatments".

This is a type of detoxification to cleanse the body. Normally the body has the innate ability to efficiently process and remove these waste materials, including the vitiated doshas. However, due to repeated dietary indiscretions, poor exercise patterns, lifestyle, and genetic predisposition the digestive enzymes, metabolic cofactors, hormones, and agnis, which regulate the body's internal homeostasis, become disorganized. This can lead to the accumulation and spread of toxins throughout the body resulting in disease. This waste matter is called ama in Ayurveda. Ama is a foul-smelling, sticky, harmful substance that needs to be completely removed from the body.

Panchakarma includes five types of treatments, which are as follows:

Vamana – Use of emetics

This therapy is mainly used in cases of chronic disorders due to Kapha dosha.

It involves induced and controlled vomiting with the help of medicines. It is used to treat chronic asthma, chronic hyperacidity, etc. It should always be administered under a physician's supervision.

Virechana – Use of laxatives

This therapy is mainly used in cases of chronic disorders due to Pitta dosha.
It involves induced and controlled purgation with the help of medicines.

Basti – Medicated enema

Involves administering medicines as enema. The medicines used can be decoctions, pure/formulated oils, milk, etc. It is used to cure arthritis, backache, etc.

Nasya – Nasal administration of medication

Nasya is administered through the nose. Medicated powders, decoctions or oil drops are introduced into the nasal passages. They remove residual doshas and toxins from the head and neck area. Nasya is used in cases of migraine, chronic rhinitis, epilepsy, etc.

Rakta Moksha – Blood-letting

Some diseases are caused by vitiation of the blood. These can be treated by letting out the vitiated blood by using leeches or syringes. It is very useful in Pitta conditions such as jaundice, ulcers, gout, piles, varicose veins, and skin diseases. This treatment must be performed by a licensed health care professional.

Panchakarma is the ultimate mind-body healing experience for detoxifying the body, strengthening the immune system, and restoring balance and well-being. It is one the most effective healing modalities in Ayurvedic medicine.

Panchakarma promotes detoxification and rejuvenation. It is recommended on a seasonal basis, as well as when an individual feels out of balance or is experiencing illness. It is also called Five Senses Therapy.

panchakarma

HOW IT WORKS

Panchakarma removes the excess doshas, corrects their imbalances and it eliminates the harmful ama from the system throughout the body's organs and channels of elimination (colon, sweat glands, lungs, bladder, urinary tract, stomach, intestines, etc). Panchakarma purifies the tissues at a very deep level. It involves daily massages and oil baths, herbal enemas, and nasal administrations. It is a very pleasurable experience. Ayurveda recommends panchakarma as a seasonal treatment for maintaining mental and physical hygiene and balance.

It is highly individualized and based on the Ayurvedic constitutional type, doshic imbalances, age, digestive strength, immune status, and many other factors. Depending on each individual's needs, all or only parts of the five therapies are utilized. Specially trained therapists must administer these procedures in a definite sequence, for a specified period of time. In addition, although panchakarma is for the most part a delightful and comfortable therapy, there can be periods of discomfort associated with the profound release of toxins. It is therefore essential that a knowledgeable expert supervise the therapy.

Like all medical procedures, panchakarma therapy always must begin with an initial consultation by a qualified Ayurvedic physician, who can determine the individual's prakriti (constitutional type), the nature of the health problem (if any), and the appropriate degree of intensity of the prescribed therapies.

TREATMENTS

The descriptions that follow cover the variety of therapies that may be performed during a Panchakarma series and represent the actual treatments used in the ancient art of life extension. Two Ayurvedic therapists working in synchrony perform many of them.

panchakarma

TREATMENTS

ABHYANGA – BENEFITS ALL THREE DOSHAS

It is an individually prepared herbal-oil massage designed to deeply penetrate the skin, relax the mind-body, break up impurities, and stimulate both arterial and lymphatic circulation. It enhances the ability of nutrients to reach starved cells and allows for the removal of stagnant waste. The desired result is a heightened state of awareness that will direct the internal healing system of the body.

SHIRODHARA

It is administered by gently and methodically pouring warm herbalized oil over the forehead, synchronizing brain waves and profoundly calming the mind, body, and spirit.

GHARSHANA

Garshana treatments consist of a dry lymphatic skin brushing with either wool or a silk glove. This enhances circulation and cleanses the skin, so that subsequent oil and herbal treatments can penetrate deeply into freshly cleansed pores of the skin.

SWEDANA

It is an individually herbalized steam bath, during which the head and the heart are kept cool while the body is heated to remove mental, emotional, and physical toxins lodged deeply within the tissues. The cool head and heart provide a sense of calm and openness, while the therapeutic steam over the entire body can penetrate and cleanse deeply, without the body becoming overheated and stressed.

PIZICHILI

It is a continuous stream of warm, herbalized oil soothingly poured over the body by two Ayurvedic therapists, as they massage the body in perfect unison. The warmth of the oil and synchronicity of the massage results in a deep tissue cleansing while supporting a heightened state of awareness that transcends description.

UDVARTANA

It is a deeply penetrating herbal paste lymphatic massage. This powerful exfoliating treatment, magically restores the skin to its natural radiance, while pressing stagnant lymphatic toxins out of the body.

BASTI

Basti is an herbal enema specially prepared to pull toxins out of the colon. This is the final stage of each daily panchakarma treatment. The freshly loosened impurities from each day of treatment are then flushed out of the body.

NASYA

Nasya consists of individually prescribed herbs and oil drops, inhaled through the nose, which clear the sinuses of excessive mucus. It is also an important therapy when medicating the central nervous system. This treatment combats the deep dryness that exists at the root of many respiratory and allergic conditions.

panchakarma

TREATMENTS

SHIRO-ABHYANGA-NASYA

It is a luxurious combination of a deep head/neck/shoulder massage and facial lymphatic massage, followed by deep inhalation of therapeutic aromatic steam and a nasal and sinus nasya with herbalized nose drops. This popular treatment is an invaluable tool balancing most head, neck, and respiratory disorders.

PINDA SWEDANA

It is a deep cleansing treatment where rice boiled in milk and herbs is massaged deeply into the tissues and joints. The treatment is deeply relaxing and rejuvenating, as well as powerfully detoxifying.

FIVE SENSES THERAPY

Five senses therapy treatment combines the therapeutic effects of all five senses working in concert. Sound therapies are specific Vedic hymns and mantras recommended for each imbalance. Touch therapy enlivens specific vital points on the body called marma points. Taste therapy uses certain herbal medicines. Sight uses Ayurvedic color therapy, and smell is accessed with combinations of rare aromatics. The effect is a harmonization of all senses bringing one's awareness to the source of thought and feeling within the heart. There are also other treatments like netra tarpana, marma massage, kati basti, karna poorana, pada dhara, hawaiian style lomi lomi, and Ayurvedic skin and beauty treatments.

SENSORY ORGANS	TREATMENTS	MOTOR ORGANS	TREATMENTS
Skin	Abhyanga (massage)	Hands	Massage, marma points
Eyes	Netrabasti, visualization anjan, netra dhara, tratak, ashchyotan	Feet	Foot massage, reflexology pad dhara
Ears	Gandharva veda music, chanting, mantra, prayer	Vocal Chords	Gargle, dhoom
Tongue	Herbal medicine, kaval, gandush	Genitals	Uttar basti
Nose	Aromatherapy, nasya, dhoom (smoke)	Anus	Basti, moola bandha

marmas

MARMAS

These vital points are the seats of life (prana). They are the junction points for tridoshas (vata, pitta, kapha), prana, tejas, ojas (subtle body) as well as sattva, rajas, and tamas.

Ayurveda describes marmas as vortex centers for muscles, blood vessels, nerves, ligaments, bone and joints. These points also represent the subtle energetic pathways of our bodies; if injured various diseases, even death, can occur. They are important pressure points on the body, like acupuncture points. Oils, herbal pastes, and kshar are applied on marmas to pacify imbalances. There are 107 primary marmas and three main marma sites—head, heart, and basti.

Marma therapy treatment is of great benefit for balancing the doshas.

AREA	VATA	PITTA	KAPHA
Head | Neck	Adhipati, Sthapani, Nila, Manya	Adhipati, Nila, Manya	Adhipati, Phana, Vidhura
Abdomen | Chest	Guda, Basti, Nabhi, Apalapa	Nabhi, Hridaya, Apstambha	Hridaya, Stanmula, Stanarohita
Hips | Back	Katikataruna, Amsa, Amsaphalaka	Kukundara, Brihati	Nitamba, Brihati, Amsaphalaka
Arms | Legs	Kshipra, Talahridya, Manibandha, Gulpha	Kurcha, Indrabasti, Kurpara (right), Janu (left)	Kshipra, Kurpara, Urvi, Janu (left)

VATA SUBDOSHAS AND MARMAS

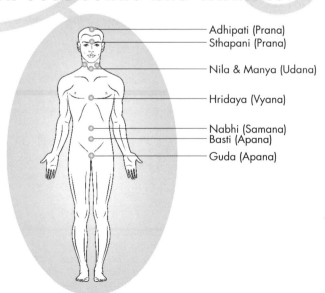

- Adhipati (Prana)
- Sthapani (Prana)
- Nila & Manya (Udana)
- Hridaya (Vyana)
- Nabhi (Samana)
- Basti (Apana)
- Guda (Apana)

marmas

PITTA SUBDOSHAS AND MARMAS

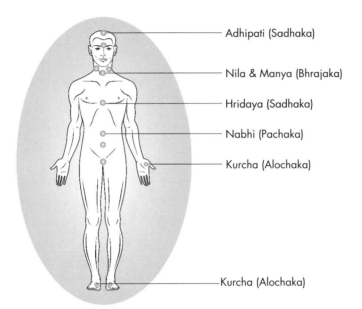

- Adhipati (Sadhaka)
- Nila & Manya (Bhrajaka)
- Hridaya (Sadhaka)
- Nabhi (Pachaka)
- Kurcha (Alochaka)
- Kurcha (Alochaka)

KAPHA SUBDOSHAS AND MARMAS

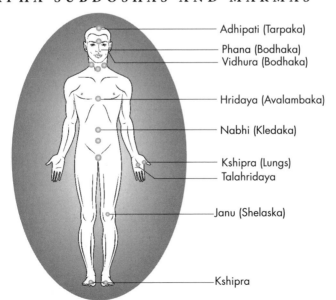

- Adhipati (Tarpaka)
- Phana (Bodhaka)
- Vidhura (Bodhaka)
- Hridaya (Avalambaka)
- Nabhi (Kledaka)
- Kshipra (Lungs)
- Talahridaya
- Janu (Shelaska)
- Kshipra

aromatherapy

AROMATHERAPY

The use of essential oils is one of the most simple and effective treatments of natural medicine.

Aromatherapy has been used since the ancient days. The Egyptians, Greeks and Arabs used aromatics 5,000 years ago for medicinal and cosmetic purposes.

In India, Ayurvedic physicians used to treat Indian royalty with dried and fresh herbs, floral waters, and aromatherapy oil for massages.

HOW IT WORKS

Aromas have a subtle energy that influences our minds, bodies and emotions.

Essential oils are of "yogavahi" property, meaning "the ability to help transport the essence of herbs to the cells and tissues of the body".

When we smell essential oils, the fragrance enters the olfactory sense (nose), stimulating the brain, which controls our desires, emotions, moods, memory, and hormones.

Due to their transdermal absorption, essential oils play an important role during the skin care treatments. Ayurveda incorporates aromatherapy into its massage oils to balance the doshas. The essential oils are not only inhaled, but also quickly absorbed by the skin into the bloodstream, and spread throughout the whole system.

Essential oils are highly concentrated essences of aromatic plants; they are not to be applied directly on the skin.

The oils are derived from different parts of the plant like flowers (jasmine), wood (sandalwood), bark (cinnamon), leaves (peppermint), roots (vetiver/khus) and fruits (lemon).

Aromatherapy

THERAPEUTIC USES

Aromatherapy is an important tool in prevention as well as in treatment.

Ayurveda offers a great variety of therapeutic aroma blends, including fumigation by burning eucalyptus leaves for the respiratory system, rose petals or saffron in the water while bathing, and burning incense sticks during meditation.

Aromatherapy can be very effective in the treatment of stress.

It stimulates or regulates the vital force prana, strengthens digestion and metabolism, and increases the immune system.

The oils help create balance through the sense of smell, and many offer targeted benefits for different subdoshas. Rose is renowned for its ability to pacify Pitta dosha. Lavender helps pacify Prana Vata, the subdosha of Vata that helps promote restful sleep.

Essential oils can be added to massage oils, facial oils, bath water, and liquid cleansers. It can also be used in homemade facials, masks, floral waters, and mists.

HOW TO USE AROMATHERAPY

Never apply essential oils directly to the skin; instead mix the recommended amounts in a base oil or in water. Test all oils for sensitivity and consult your physician before using essential oils if you are pregnant, nursing, or have a medical condition.

DOSHA	RECOMMENDED ESSENTIAL OILS
Vata	Lavender, Cedar wood, Sage, Geranium, Tulasi, Juniper.
Pitta	Sandalwood, Rose, Lotus, Jasmine, Gardena, Vetiver, Peppermint, Lemon.
Kapha	Eucalyptus, Tulsi, Basil, Camphor, Sage, Rosemary.

HERBS

HERBS FOR HEALTH AND HEALING
Herbs have tremendous healing powers.

Herbs have specific effects on the physical body. Each herb has its own intelligence, targeting specific areas of the body with precision. Herbs regulate your bodily functions, cleanse, and nourish the human body.

The goal of Ayurveda is prevention, preservation, and rejuvenation of the body.

By using Ayurvedic herbal medicines you ensure all these functions without side effects. Ayurvedic herbs are inhaled, applied on wounds directly, or administered orally depending on your requirement. They are used according to their energetics and each dravya (herb) has five categories (qualifications). They are rasa, veerya, vipaka, prabhava, and karma.

RASA
Ra-taste, relish or praise | sa-juice, sap or secretion

Rasa is the taste or sensation that the tongue experiences as soon as it comes into contact with food. There are six tastes and each one is made up of two of the five elements. Rasa also has an effect on pacifying or aggravating the doshas.

TASTE	ELEMENTS	VATA	PITTA	KAPHA
Madhura	Sweet	Earth + Water	↓	↓	↑
Amla	Sour	Earth + Fire	↓	↑	↑
Lavana	Salty	Water + Fire	↓	↑	↑
Katu	Pungent	Fire + Air	↑	↑	↓
Tikta	Bitter	Air + Ether	↑	↓	↓
Kashaya	Astringent	Air + Earth	↑	↓	↓

The Energetics of herbs

VEERYA
Potency, energy, strength

It is the energy of an herb that is released when ingested. The release of energy can be sheeta (cooling) or ushna (heating).

TYPE	
Sheeta Cooling V↑ P↓ K↑	**Action** – strengthens, tones dhatus. Refreshes the body, slows agni, reduces irritation and inflammation. **Rasa** – sweet, astringent, and bitter. **Examples** – aloe vera and lotus.
Ushna Heating V↓ P↑ K↓	**Action** – balances Kapha and Vata. Improves circulation, helps digestion, promotes sweating, and ignites agni. **Rasa** – sour, salty, and pungent. **Examples** – dry ginger, pippali, and chitrak.

VIPAKA
Post-Digestive Effect

Vipaka is the post-digestive effect of food on the body. Ayurveda explains that there are three stages of digestion. In each stage, a post-digestive taste has a special and unique effect upon the different dhatus. There are three types of vipaka.

VIPAKA	
Madhura Sweet	**Taste** – sweet and salty **Effects** – helps eliminate malas, promotes dhatus growth, increases Kapha.
Amla Sour	**Taste** – sour **Effects** – strengthens agni, decreases ama and Vata, increases Pitta.
Katu Pungent	**Taste** – pungent, astringent and bitter **Effects** – blocks and causes constipation, increases body excretions, increases Vata.

the energetics of herbs

PRABHAVA
*It is the special and unique power of an herb that has
a variable action.*

It is unique as it does not fit in the category of other herbs that present the same rasa, veerya or vipaka. A good example of prabhava can be found in comparing the herbs danti and chitrak. They both present pungent rasa and vipaka, and heating veerya. Danti is laxative and chitrak is not.

KARMA
Action

Herbs are classified in accordance to their particular therapeutic action. There are various types of herb classifications according to Ayurveda.

HERB TYPE	
Deepana (Stimulant herbs)	**Action** – stimulates agni, digests ama, increases appetite. **Examples** Aajwyan, black pepper, pippali.
Pachana (Digestive herbs)	**Action** – helps digestion. **Examples** Chitrak, ginger, vidanga.
Shodhana (Purification herbs)	**Action** – purifies and cleanses body; decreases Pitta and Kapha, and increases Vata. **Examples** Haritaki, castor oil.
Anuloman (Carminative herbs)	**Action** – normalizes Vata, promotes digestion, and relieves gastrointestinal pain and distention. **Examples** Cooling – fennel, cardamom, coriander. Heating – ajwayan, cumin, garlic.
Virechana (Purgative herbs)	**Action** – promotes elimination of toxins from the intestinal walls, forces bowel movement. **Examples** Castor oil, senna.

The Energetics of herbs

HERBAL DOSE AND TIME OF INTAKE

The dosage of an herb varies according to certain factors such as age, constitution, type of disease, and the person's strength. As for the time of administration, Ayurveda enforces the importance of taking the herbs at a certain time of the day, so the herb has a better and more efficient effect. The best time to administer the herbs are:

EARLY IN THE MORNING (ON AN EMPTY STOMACH)

Reduces Kapha conditions and mucus.

BEFORE MEALTIME

Decreases Vata conditions. Stimulates the colon and lower part of the body (apana vayu).

DURING MEALTIME

Improves digestion, affects the stomach and small intestine.

AFTER MEALTIME

Strengthens the lungs and works in the upper part of the body.

TAKEN FREQUENTLY

For acute conditions, cough, asthma, breathlessness, vomiting.

BEDTIME

For sleep disorders.

ANUPANA
Carrier

Herbal medicines are prescribed with various mediums of intake or carriers, such as hot water, milk, honey, etc. Anupana enhances the therapeutic effect, and deepens the effect targeting different organs. Some anupanas according to the doshas are:

DOSHA	QUALITIES	EXAMPLES
VATA	Moist, warm	Sesame oil, warm water
PITTA	Cool and sweet	Ghee, cool water, milk
KAPHA	Dry and warm	Honey, warm water

important Herbs

TEN IMPORTANT HERBS

AMALAKI (Embilica officinalis)

Action – rejuvenative, aphrodisiac, laxative, hemostatic, tonic.

Uses – all Pitta diseases, arthritis, asthma, fever, gastritis, hemorrhoids, insomnia, vertigo.

Effect on dosha – V ↓ P ↓ K ↑   **Energetics** – all tastes except salty-cold-sweet

ASHWAGANDHA (Withenia somnifera)

Action – rejuvenative, aphrodisiac, nervine, analgesic, sedative.

Uses – anxiety, brain tonic, age preventive, blood pressure, fatigue, urinary diseases.

Effect on dosha – V ↓ P ↑ K ↓   **Energetics** – astringent/bitter-hot-sweet

BRAHMI | GOTU KOLA (Bacopa Moniera) | Tridoshic

Action – diuretic, nervine, rejuvenative.

Uses – asthma, cough, blood purifier, immune system booster; brain, and nerves.

Effect on dosha – V ↓ P ↓ K ↓   **Energetics** – bitter-cold-sweet

GUDUCHI (Tinosphora Cardifolia) | Tridoshic

Action – alterative, anti-aging, anti-pyretic, diuretic.

Uses – immune booster, digestion, constipation, skin disease, blood purifier.

Effect on dosha – V ↓ P ↓ K ↓   **Energetics** – bitter/sweet-hot-sweet

HARITAKI (Terminelia Chebula)

Action – rejuvenative, laxative, nervine, expectorant, tonic.

Uses – cough, asthma, gas, vomiting, nervous disorders, indigestion, memory.

Effect on dosha – V ↓ P ↓ K ↓   **Energetics** – all except salty-hot-sweet

important Herbs

TEN IMPORTANT HERBS

KUMARI | ALOE VERA (Aloe barbadensis)

Action – rejuvenative, alterative, digestive, purgative, tonic.

Uses – colds, lung diseases, intestinal worms, hemorrhoids, blood tonic, burns, herpes, skin diseases.

Effect on dosha – V ↓ P ↓ K ↓   **Energetics** – sweet/cold/sweet

---

MANJISHTA (Rubia cordifolia)

Action – alterative, astringent, diuretic, hemostatic.

Uses – blood circulation, cleanses liver, edema, hepatitis, menstruation, menopause, skin problems.

Effect on dosha – V ↑ P ↓ K ↓   **Energetics** – pungent/ bitter/astringent-cold-pungent

---

MUSTA | NUTGRASS (Cyperus rotundus)

Action – alterative, antifungal, carminative, diuretic, stimulant.

Uses – menstrual disorders, gastritis, indigestion, malabsorption, vomiting, palpitation.

Effect on dosha – V ↓ P ↓ K ↑   **Energetics** – pungent/ bitter/astringent-cold-pungent

---

NEEM (Azadirecta indica)

Action – alterative, bitter tonic, antiseptic, anti-emetic, antibiotic.

Uses – blood purifier, inflammation of muscles and joints, cleanses liver, parasites, skin disorders.

Effect on dosha – V ↑ P ↓ K ↓   **Energetics** – bitter/astringent-cold-pungent

---

SHATAVARI (Asperagus recemosus)

Action – nutritive, diuretic, tonic, aphrodisiac, antispasmodic.

Uses – cough, diarrhea, immune system, female reproductive system, menopause, ulcers, fevers.

Effect on dosha – V ↓ P ↓ K ↑   **Energetics** – sweet/bitter-cold-sweet

Disease Diagnosis and Management

SIX STAGES OF DISEASE MANIFESTATION
SHAT KRIYA KAL

Sanchaya	Accumulation
Prakopa	Aggravation
Prasara	Dissemination
Sthana sanshraya	Localization
Vyakti	Manifestation
Bheda	Differentiation

FIVE FOLD DISEASE ASSESSMENT
NIDAN PANCHAK

Nidan	Causative factors
Purvaroopa	Initial symptoms
Roopa	Symptoms
Upashaya	Aid used to eradicate disease
Samprapti	Pathogenesis

AYURVEDIC PATIENT EXAMINATION
TRI VIDH (TRIFOLD EXAMINATION)

Darshana	To see
Sparshana	To touch
Prashna	To ask questions

Disease Diagnosis and Management

ASHTA VIDHA
(EIGHT FOLD PATIENT EXAMINATION)

EXAMINATION OF THE COMPLEXION | AKRITI PARIKSHA

The disease is diagnosed by reading the physical features of the face.

EXAMINATION OF THE EYES | DRIKA PARIKSHA

Color, shape, and size helps with the diagnosis of imbalances.

EXAMINATION OF THE SPEECH AND VOICE | SHABDA PARIKSHA

The balanced doshas produce a natural and healthy voice. The aggravated dosha makes different sounds.

EXAMINATION OF THE TONGUE | JIVHA PARIKSHA

The state of the digestive system is also assessed by the condition of the tongue.

EXAMINATION OF THE SKIN | SPARSHA PARIKSHA

It is used for assessing the state of organs and tissues, with the help of palpation, by obtaining information about temperature, texture, and tenderness.

EXAMINATION OF THE STOOL | MALA PARIKSHA

There are various references of color, smell, and consistency of stool in different diseases. The stool carries a foul odor and sinks in water, if there is poor digestion and absorption of food.

EXAMINATION OF URINE | MUTRA PARIKSHA

It is usually done by examining the sample of urine and questioning the patient. Oil drops are used for further examination of urine.

EXAMINATION OF THE PULSE | NADI PARIKSHA

With the help of just three fingers you detect the balance or imbalances in the physical and mental state of one's health.

FUNDAMENTALS OF AYURVEDIC CHIKITSA/TREATMENTS

AYURVEDIC PATIENT EXAMINATION

The treatment of disease can be classified as:

Shamana therapy (palliative treatment)

Shodhana therapy (purification treatment)

Pathya Apathya (dietary do's and don't recommendations)

Nidan Parivarjan (avoidance of disease; causing and aggravating factors)

Satvavajaya (psychotherapy)

Rasayana therapy (use of immune modulators and rejuvenation medicines)

YOGA

yoga principles

WHAT IS YOGA?

The word yoga is derived from the Sanskrit word 'Yuja' meaning to unite, combine or integrate.

The union of the 'Atma' with the 'Parmatma', the finite with the infinite. A state of integration between the individual consciousness and cosmic consciousness, or a total integration of the physical, mental, and spiritual aspects of the human being.

It has also other meanings such as:

Yogaha chitta vritti nirodhaha – control of fluctuations of the mind.

Yogaha karmasu kaushalyam – proficiency in the work.

Yoga of herbs – combination of herbal formulas.

Yoga of planets – a specific combination of the grahas (planets) in Vedic astrology.

The aim of yoga is to prepare the body to achieve the tranquility of mind that is necessary for the realization of the Divine or Supreme.

The practice of yoga is a simple process of synchronizing one's breath with movement into various physical postures. The combination of these two elements is what makes yoga unique and highly therapeutic. In order to heal the body, one must work with its counterpart, the mind, and see the correlation between the two in order to truly address the cause of disease.

In this way, yoga is a profound method for healing the root causes of illness, leading to a lasting feeling of peace and happiness.

The practice of yoga goes back an estimated 5,000 years. The sage Patanjali compiled the Yoga Sutras, a philosophical guide based on the Vedas. The Yoga Sutras include a wide range of yogic practices such as asanas, pranayama, meditation, and mantras. It also delineates the eight limbs of yoga to aid in the development of consciousness. They help with our journey from the outer world to the inner self toward the final goal in reaching Samadhi (liberation).

They are:

Yamas – social conduct

Niyamas – behavior

Asana – body postures

Pranayama – control of breath

Pratyahara – control of senses

Dharana – concentration

Dhyani – meditation

Samadhi – union

yoga

PATHS OF YOGA

There are many paths of Yoga offering many methods. One should follow the path that most speaks to the heart and fits one's nature best. Some of the Yogic paths are Jnana Yoga, Bhakti Yoga, Kriya Yoga, Karma Yoga, Hatha Yoga, Raja Yoga.

YOGA	
Jnana Yoga	the search of knowledge and truth
Bhakti Yoga	the practice of devotion to the Divine
Kriya Yoga	the practice of techniques
Karma Yoga	the path of service
Hatha Yoga	the path of effort
Raja Yoga	integral yoga

WHAT DOES HATHA MEAN?
Ha means "sun" and tha means "moon".

Hatha yoga, from where the physical postures derived, has its basic principles acquired from tantra. Hatha believes in the creation of balance and union between opposites: masculine and feminine, hot and cool, sun and moon within us. Hatha also means forceful and willful, while yoga means union. It takes discipline and effort to harmonize and unify opposites (body and soul). Sequences of asanas are designed to transform the physical body to achieve enlightenment. The postures' purpose also aims to open the channels of the body (nadis), releasing energy to flow freely.

YOGA AND AYURVEDA

Yoga is greatly incorporated in Ayurveda, as they complement each other in the preservation of mind, body, and soul.

The practice of asanas, pranyama, prattyahara, dharana, dhyani, marmas, carefully chosen according to Prakriti, will improve physical vitality, calm the mind, balance doshas, and bring inner peace.

The recommendation of a Yoga path will depend upon the individual, age, character, and constitutional type in order to obtain an ideal therapeutic effect.

The Mind

THE FOUR FUNCTIONS OF MIND

According to Ayurveda principles, observing and discriminating between the four functions of mind is a very important part of Yoga meditation.

They are:

	FUNCTIONS
Manas I Mind	Outer mind, sensations
Ahankara I Ego	Ego identity
Buddhi I Intellect	Inner knowledge
Chitta I Memory	Self, core mind

THE THREE GUNAS OR QUALITIES
Sattva, Raja, Tamas

There are three universal qualities, or forces, in nature. These forces are always present in different proportions within mind, body and soul.

GUNAS	
Sattva	Harmony, balance, order, stability, clarity, purity
Raja	Dynamic, energetic, changeable
Tamas	Inert, heavy, negative, lethargic, dull

THE TRIGUNAS AND THE DOSHAS

GUNAS	VATA	PITTA	KAPHA
Sattvic	Flexible, enthusiastic, positive, adaptable	Independent, clear, perceptive, discriminating, a leader	Peaceful, stable, receptive, nurturing, loving
Rajasic	Indecisive, fearful, restless, nervous, agitated	Impulsive, ambitious, proud, angry, judgmental	Attached, materialistic, greedy, possessive
Tamasic	Depressed, fearful, addictive, disturbed	Offensive, wicked, vindictive, destructive	Lethargic, dull, slow, apathetic

the three bodies

PHYSICAL, SUBTLE, CAUSAL BODIES

TYPE	PHYSICAL | STHOOLA	SUBTLE | SUKSHAMA	CAUSAL | KARANA
Composition	Gross elements	Subtle elements	Causal elements
State	Waker	Dreamer	Deep Sleeper
Guna	Tamas	Raja	Sattva
Identity	Body	Mind	Soul

the five sheaths

FIVE KOSHAS OR SHEATHS

KOSHA	
Annamaya (Food sheath)	Sustains the body. Composed of the five elements.
Pranamaya (Breath sheath)	Energizes the body and mind. Composed of five pranas and the five motor organs.
Manomaya (Mental sheath)	Process of thoughts and emotions. Composed of mind and five sense organs.
Gyanamaya (Intellectual sheath)	Responsible for thinking and discrimination. Composed of intelligence and reason.
Anandamaya (Bliss sheath)	Love and consciousness. Bliss and gunas.

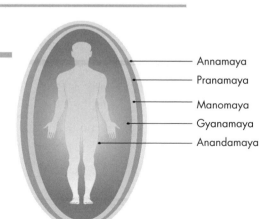

Annamaya
Pranamaya
Manomaya
Gyanamaya
Anandamaya

The subtle body

CHAKRAS

Chakras or wheels of light are seven subtle energy centers aligned along the spinal column in which energy flows in a non-physical way between body, mind, and soul.

NAME	PETALS	MEANING	LOCATION	VAYU	BEEJ	COLOR
Mooladhara	4	Root	Perineum	Apana	Lam	Red
Swadhisthana	6	Self-abode	Genitals	Apana	Vam	Orange
Manipura	10	City of gems	Navel	Samana	Ram	Yellow
Anahata	12	Unstruck sound	Heart	Vyana	Yam	Green
Vishuddha	16	Very pure	Throat	Udana	Ham	Blue
Ajna	2	Command	Third-eye	Prana	Ksham	Indigo
Sahasrara	1,000	1,000 petals lotus	Top of head	All	Om	Violet

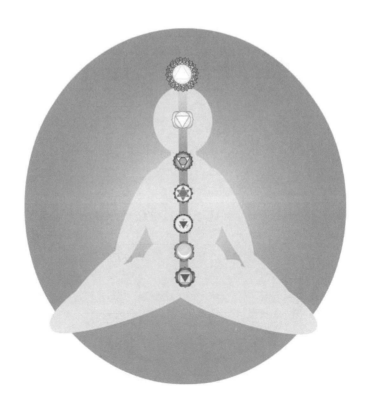

asana and the doshas

TYPES OF ASANAS

Ayurveda recommends that for an optimum practice of asanas one should always consider the individual constitution and address the seven main types of postures.

STANDING

Improves posture and benefits legs and hips. Increases mobility in shoulder and neck.

BALANCING

Improves concentration, coordination, body posture. It creates heat in the body.

SEATED

Benefits the spine and improves flexibility to hips, knees, and ankles.

INVERTED

Anytime the legs are in higher position than the heart. This posture improves circulation and it strengthens the upper body.

FORWARD BENDS

Benefits lower back, spine, shoulders, and neck and releases tension from the abdominal area.

BACK BENDS

Opens the chest and lungs, hips and shoulders, and improves the stability of the spine.

TWISTING

Twisting postures increase mobility in the shoulder and hip areas. Increase spine flexibility and are also beneficial in releasing stiffness and tension.

surya namaskara | sun salutation

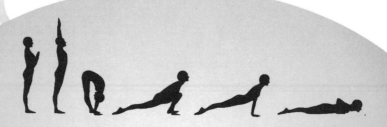

asana and the doshas

POSTURES FOR THE DOSHAS

VATA ASANAS	PITTA ASANAS	KAPHA ASANAS
Mountain pose Tadasana	Downward dog pose Adhomukha svanasana	Tree pose Vrikshasana
Triangle pose Trikonasana	Spread legs forward bend pose Padottanasana	Warrior pose Virabhadrasana
Boat pose Navasana	Full forward bend pose Paschimottanasana	Peacock pose Mayurasana
Shoulder stand pose Sarvangasana	Inverted action pose Viparita karani	Headstand pose Shirsasana
Head to knee Janu shirasana	Child's pose Balasana	Cobra Bhujangasana
Full forward bend pose Paschimottanasana	Perfect sitting pose Siddhasana	Boat pose Navasana
Sage twist pose Marichyasana	Seated spinal twist pose Ardha matsyendrasana	Open legs forward bend pose Upavistha konasana

surya namaskara | sun salutation

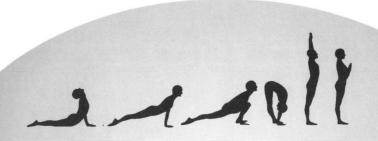

pranayama

WHAT IS PRANAYAMA AND HOW DOES IT WORK?

"Prana" means life force and "Aayama" means to regulate or enhance breathing efficiency. The main purpose of Pranayama is to slow down the respiratory rate and infuse prana in the subtle nadis.

Prana activates the dormant psychic energy called "Kundalini", which resides at the base of spine near mooladhara chakra. Prana energetically stimulates Kundalini for its ascension toward higher chakras.

When sufficient, fire Yoga is generated within the system, the Ajna chakra sends a feedback to the base (the mooladhara) of kundalini and the dormant potential energy is awakened to increase the energy flow to the Ajna chakra. This is the purpose of pranayama.

The science of pranayama is based on the retention of prana called 'kumbhaka'. Inhalation (poorak) and exhalation (rechak) are merely incidental. Those who are serious in awakening the hidden recesses of the brain need to perfect the art of retention (kumbhaka). During kumbhaka there is an increased blood flow into the brain and simultaneously heat is generated in the system.

WHEN TO PERFORM PRANAYAMA

Pranayama yoga must be performed on an empty stomach. The best time for practice is the early morning, preferably before sunrise, when the pollution is at its lowest level and the body and brain are still free. However, if morning is unsuitable, pranayama may be practiced after sunset, when the air is cool and pleasant.

pranayama

MAJOR TYPES OF PRANAYAMA

NADI SODHANA | ALTERNATE NOSTRIL BREATHING

Cleanses the lunar and solar channels (ida and pingala) and calms the mind.

KAPALABHATI PRANAYAMA | SHINING SKULL

Cleanses respiratory passages and calms the mind. Massages all digestive organs.

UJJAYI PRANAYAMA | CONQUERING BREATH

Releases mental and nervous stress, and cleanses channels.

BHASTRIKA PRANAYAMA | BELLOWS BREATH

Strengthens the heart, lungs, and immune system. Improves digestion and calms the mind.

BHRAMARI PRANAYAMA | HUMMING BEE BREATH

Relieves stress, tension, and helps with sleep.

BAHYA PRANAYAMA

Benefits the digestive system and enhances concentration.

SHITALI PRANAYAMA | COOLING BREATH

Decreases heat, burning and heat sensations.

SHITKARI PRANAYAMA | HISSING BREATH

Benefits gum and teeth.

BENEFITS OF PRANAYAMA

Improves concentration and clarity of thought.

Increases mental and physical endurance.

Deepens relaxation, meditation, and is a scientific method of controlling breath.

Provides complete relaxation to the nervous system.

Provides relief from pain caused by the compression of nerves.

Helps to increase oxygen supply to the brain, which in turn helps to control the mind.

Mudras

MUDRAS

The physical body is made up of five elements ether, air, water, fire and earth.

Imbalance of these elements disrupts the immune system and causes disease.

Deficiencies in any of these elements can be corrected by connecting one part of the body with another in a particular manner through mudras.

When a finger representing one element is brought into contact with the thumb, that element is balanced.

Mudras start electromagnetic currents within the body, which balance various elements and restore health. The joining of fingers creates an effect on the human body.

FIVE FINGERS FOR FIVE ELEMENTS

Thumb | Ether

Index | Air

Middle | Fire

Ring | Water

Little | Earth

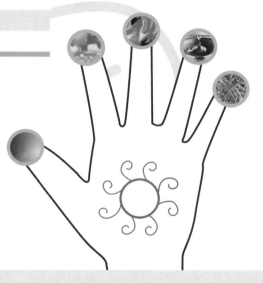

WHEN TO PRACTICE MUDRA

It can be practiced any time preferably in a comfortable position.

Mudra can be practiced in the beginning for at least four to five minutes a day. Once you built strength, it can be practiced up to 30 minutes. If a mudra cannot be made in both hands, you may do it in one hand only.

Mudras

DIFFERENT TYPES OF MUDRAS

MUDRAS	
Gyan Mudra (Knowledge)	**Benefits** – Purifies the mind and sharpens memory. **Method** – Join the tip of the thumb and index finger, keep the other three fingers stretched out.
Shoonya Mudra (Emptiness)	**Benefits** – Relieves ear pain and diseases. **Method** – Press the middle finger down with the thumb and keep the other three fingers straight.
Apana Mudra (Digestion)	**Benefits** – Helps to clear the body by eliminating waste matter. **Method** – Join the tip of the thumb with the tip of middle and ring finger, keep the other fingers straight.
Prana Mudra (Life)	**Benefits** – Improves the life force throughout the body. **Method** – Join the tip of the thumb with the tips of little and ring finger; keeping the other two fingers straight.
Vayu Mudra (Air)	**Benefits** – Helps in diseases related to air imbalance. **Method** – Press the index finger on the base of thumb and keep the other three fingers stretched out.
Prithvi Mudra (Earth)	**Benefits** – Strengthens the body. **Method** – Join the tip of the thumb and ring finger, keep the other three fingers stretched out.
Varuna Mudra (Water)	**Benefits** – Balances water content in the body and refreshes the body. **Method** – Join the tip of the thumb and little finger, keep the other three fingers stretched out.
Surya Mudra (Sun)	**Benefits** – Helps reduce heaviness in the body. **Method** – Bend the ring finger and press down with the thumb, keep the other three fingers stretched out.
Ling Mudra (Heat)	**Benefits** – Produces heat in the body and helps in relieving cold and cough. **Method** – Interlock the fingers of both hands together. Keeping the left thumb up (encircled by right thumb and index finger) i.e. left thumb should be vertically straight and right thumb around it.

mudras

MUDRAS	
Gyan Mudra (Knowledge)	
Shoonya Mudra (Emptiness)	
Apana Mudra (Digestion)	
Prana Mudra (Life)	
Vayu Mudra (Air)	

MUDRAS	
Prithvi Mudra (Earth)	
Varuna Mudra (Water)	
Surya Mudra (Sun)	
Ling Mudra (Heat)	

Bandhas

BANDHAS
The word bandha means to lock, to tie together.

The use of bandhas in Yoga is very important as it helps in the cleansing process of the body and the flow of energy. During the process of practicing bandhas certain areas are locked in a particular manner.

There are three main bandha techniques that involve three muscle groups: cervical (neck) muscles, abdominal muscles and perineal muscles. These three bandhas, when used together, are called Maha Bandha or the great lock.

The practice of bandhas should be taught and supervised by an experienced teacher.

Bandhas

BANDHAS	
Jalandhar Bandha	Jalan means net and dhar means stream or flow. **Benefits** All doshas. Improves voice quality, throat disorders, mental clarity, stimulates brain function. **Region** Neck and upper spine.
Uddiyana Bandha	Uddiyana means to rise up or to fly upward. **Benefits** All doshas. Reverses aging, tones heart region, nerves, glands, and muscles. Improves vitality, and increases oxygen absorption in the brain. **Region** Diaphragm and pelvic floor.
Mula Bandha	Mula means root, firmly fixed, source, or cause. **Benefits** All doshas. Balances hormones, improves digestion, blood circulation, and nervous system functions. **Region** Navel and pelvic floor.

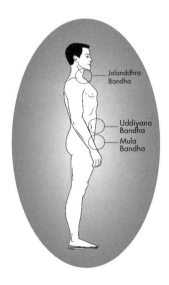

Jalanddhra Bandha

Uddiyana Bandha

Mula Bandha

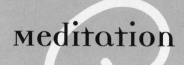

meditation

WHAT IS MEDITATION?

Meditation is derived from two latin words: meditari (to contemplate) and mederi (to heal). Both of these words are derived from the Sanskrit word medha (wisdom or pure intellect). Meditation simply means awareness and mindfulness.

Meditation is an effortless technique that is simple and highly effective to manage stress on a daily basis. With a little practice one can cultivate a state of mind, which can be directed inward in order to feel calm and flexible for your external needs.

It helps to calm your mind and become more focused. Fifteen to twenty minutes of breathing or mantra meditation will help to reduce stress and reestablish inner peace and well-being.

Meditation also helps to understand the tendency of your own mind. One can learn how to transform negative thoughts into positive affirmations. It is not religious, but a spiritual practice that improves the quality and quantity of human life.

HEALTH BENEFITS OF MEDITATION

BENEFITS
Lowers oxygen consumption. Decreases respiratory rate.
Increases blood flow and slows the heart rate. Increases exercise tolerance in heart patients. Good for people with high blood pressure.
Decreases muscle tension (any pain due to tension) and headaches.
Reduces anxiety attacks by lowering blood lactate levels. Increases serotonin production, which influences mood and behavior.
Builds self-confidence. Leads to a deeper level of relaxation.
Helps in chronic diseases like allergies, arthritis, etc.
Helps in post-operative healing.
Reduces pre-menstrual syndrome.
Enhances the immune system. Research has revealed that meditation increases activity of 'natural-killer cells', which fight bacteria and cancer cells.

meditation benefits

HEALTH BENEFITS FOR WOMEN

Women's nervous systems are very sensitive and vulnerable to emotional ups and downs. Every month, women's bodies experience hormonal changes, which affect the state of mind. Meditation practice for women slows down the emotional fluctuations. It improves resilience and decision-making skills. Daily meditation practices will improve overall energy, mental clarity, emotional stability, and increase happiness and joy.

HEALTH BENEFITS FOR MOTHERS-TO-BE

Meditation for expectant mothers is a wonderful way to connect with their baby. It is a mindful exercise, which sends loving, healing energy to the baby for its growth and well being. Meditation during all the trimesters helps balance doshas and dhatus and fosters a sattvic mind for both mother and baby.

Meditation during pregnancy enlivens their state of consciousness and creates emotional stability for a healthy and productive life.

MEDITATION TECHNIQUES

Many techniques are available for effective meditation.

Even though various meditation techniques are used in different cultures, meditation is universal. Some techniques use concentration, others allows for the free flow of thoughts and their observations. Presented below are some samples of the common meditation. Meditation should be learned under the guidance of a teacher.

MANTRA MEDITATION

Specific sounds are repeated (japa) to achieve a meditative state.

TRATAKA MEDITATION | TO GAZE STEADILY

A steady gaze is placed onto an object.

sanskrit

SANSKRIT

Sanskrit is the world's most ancient language. It is considered to be the mother of all Indo-European languages. The word Sanskrit simply means "created to perfection." It is usually referred to as "Deva Vaani" or language of gods, and the Sanskrit script is called "Deva Naagari".

It is a phonetic language and the words are pronounced exactly the way they are written. Sanskrit is arranged in a very scientific manner with regard to its alphabet, grammar, and vocabulary. It is the language of the Vedas. All Vedic scriptures like Ayurveda, Yoga, Jyotish, Upanishads were all written in Sanskrit and were passed down to Vedic families through oral transmission and memorization.

It is a sacred language of cosmic consciousness and light. Sanskrit sounds, when recited properly, have calming as well as stimulating effects on the physiology. All the 50 letters of the alphabet are correlated with the chakras and the pranic body. Recent research has shown that Sanskrit mantras activate and trigger neurons in the brain, and restructure the neural pathways between the brain's two hemispheres, enlivening higher states of consciousness.

sanskrit alphabet

Independent Vowel Signs	अ a	आ ā	इ i	ई ī	उ u	ऊ ū	
			ए e	ऐ ai	ओ o	औ au	
	ऋ ṛ	ॠ ṝ	ऌ ḷ		अं aṅ/añ/an/aṃ		अः aḥ
Guttural	क ka	ख kha	ग ga	घ gha	ङ ṅa		
Palatal	च ca	छ cha	ज ja	झ jha	ञ ña		
Cerebral	ट ṭa	ठ ṭha	ड ḍa	ढ ḍha	ण ṇa		
Dental	त ta	थ tha	द da	ध dha	न na		
Labial	प pa	फ pha	ब ba	भ bha	म ma		
Semi-vowels	य ya	र ra	ल la	व va			
Aspirate & Sibilants	श śa	ष ṣa	स sa	ह ha		क्ष kṣa	ज्ञ jña

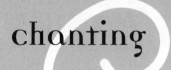

chanting

WHAT IS CHANTING?

Chanting involves repeating a mantra or a prayer. "Man" means mind and "tra" means across, so a mantra is something that is repeatedly crossing the mind to control thoughts for meditation.

Chanting is a process of connecting with the heart and soul. While chanting, the mind is given something to play with, helping it to calm down. It also allows one to bypass the mind to get to the heart.

Repeating mantras out loud has a specific effect on the body. During the mantra recitation, the tongue hits meridian points on the top of the upper palate of the mouth, which affects the energies travelling to different glands in the body. As these meridian points are stimulated, one is physically producing the effect of relaxation and an altered state of consciousness.

ORIGIN OF MANTRAS

Mantras are believed to have originated in the Vedic scriptures. These teachings contain thousands of mantras that were received by the Rishis from the Cosmic Mind. Mantras carry a certain pure vibrational power and sound, so using the proper pronunciation is very important.

Mantras can be repeated mentally or chanted, and are a very powerful tool in healing the physical and subtle body, mind, and soul. They can be used to calm the mind, to treat tension, and to restore emotional balance.

OM is the most important of all mantras. OM is the original vibration that all other mantras are derived from. All mantras generally begin and often also end with OM.

THE POWER OF SOUND

The sound of a mantra can lift a person toward a higher consciousness. In the recitation of Sanskrit mantras, the sound is very important, for it can transform, while leading to power and strength.

Different sounds have different effects on the human psyche.

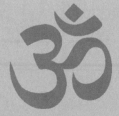

Mantras

IMPORTANT MANTRAS

Gayatri Mantra (Goddess mantra)

Gayatri Mantra (the mother of the Vedas), the foremost mantra in Hinduism and Hindu beliefs, inspires wisdom. Its literal meaning is "May the Almighty God illuminate our intellect to lead us along the righteous path." The mantra is also a prayer to the "giver of light and life" – the sun (Savitur).

Aum Bhoor Bhuwah Swaha
Tat Savitur Varenyam
Bhargo Devasaya Dheemahi
Dhiyo Yo Naha Prachodayat.

Ganesh mantra (for wisdom or knowledge)

Om Gam Ganapatayae Namah

The Maha Mrityunjaya Mantra (Great death conquering mantra)

Aum Tryambakam yajamahe
Sugandhim pushti-vardhanam
Urvarukamiva bandhanan
Mrityor mukshiya mamritat''

Surya Namaskara (Sun Salutation)

Surya Namaskar is the Salutation to the Sun, the energy provider.
Surya Namaskar has postures that goes with each particular mantra.

Om Mitraaya Namah	Salutations to the friend of all
Om Ravaye Namah	Salutations to the shining one
Om Sooryaya Namah	Salutations to the dispeller of darkness
Om Bhaanave Namah	Salutations to the one who illuminates
Om Khagaaya Namah	Salutations to the one who moves
Om Pooshne Namah	across the sky
Om Hiranya Garbhaaya Namah	Salutations to the giver of strength
Om Marichaya Namah	Salutations to the golden cosmic self
Om Aadityaaya Namah	Salutations to the rays of the sun
Om Savitre Namah	Salutations to the son Aditi, the infinite
Om Arkaaya Namah	cosmic mother
Om Bhaaskaraya Namah	Salutations to the stimulating power
Om Sri Savitra Soorya	Salutations to the remover of afflictions
Narayanaaya Namah	Salutations to the one who leads to enlightenment

vedic branches

vedic astrology
jyotish

jyotish principles
charts
rashis, grahas and bhavas
dashas and gochara

vedic architecture
vaastu

vaastu principles

music
gandharva veda

music principles

Jyotish

WHAT IS JYOTISH OR VEDIC ASTROLOGY?

"Jyotish" is a Sanskrit word that is derived from two roots, "Jyoti" and "Isha", which respectively mean, "Light" and "Divine".

Jyotish is commonly referred as Vedic Astrology. It is a science of light, both the light of celestial bodies and the internal light of the soul (jeevatman), which unfolds the knowledge of how the planets and stars influence an individual human life and general mundane events. Jyotish also sheds light on individual "karma" or destiny.

Jyotish is predictive astrology. It uses accurate astronomical data (Sidhanta) and mathematical calculations to determine the positions of the planets in relation to the Earth at the time of birth, in order to foretell (Hora) the future events of a person's life. Jyotish is about understanding how to best perform in time. It is a behavior analysis and forecasting system, based on astronomical calculations, that assist in anticipating the benefits and challenges that lie ahead. Vedic astrology advises how to modify actions for a better outcome. So while one might naturally have the will to take the action, Jyotish prepares the individual in the best possible way.

HOW DOES JYOTISH OR VEDIC ASTROLOGY DIFFER FROM WESTERN ASTROLOGY?

Western astrology, or Tropical astrology, emphasizes the relationship of the Sun to the Earth and the seasons. The Vedic astrology is based on the Sidereal Zodiac and the planets' movements are tracked against fixed observable stars in the sky.

Another difference is that the Western astrological year starts in Aries, and the Vedic starts in Pisces. More emphasis is also placed on the Moon than the Sun.

Vedic astrology considers the rising sign, or ascendant, more important than the Sun. The ascendant is represented by the sign on the eastern horizon at the time of birth, and it changes every two hours. Below is a comparison chart between Vedic and Western astrological year.

RASHI I SIGN	VEDIC CALENDAR	WESTERN CALENDAR
Mesha I Aries	Apr 13–May 14	Mar 21–Apr 19
Vrishabha I Taurus	May 15–Jun 14	Apr 20–May 20
Mithuna I Gemini	Jun 15–Jul 14	May 21–Jun 20
Karka I Cancer	Jul 15–Aug 14	Jun 21–Jul 22
Simha I Leo	Aug 15–Sep 15	Jul 23–Aug 22
Kanya I Virgo	Sep 16–Oct 15	Aug 23–Sept 22
Tula I Libra	Oct 16–Nov 14	Sept 23–Oct 22
Vrishika I Scorpio	Nov 15–Dec 14	Oct 23–Nov 21
Dhanus I Sagittarius	Dec 15–Jan 13	Nov 22–Dec 21
Makara I Capricorn	Jan 14–Feb 12	Dec 22–Jan 19
Kumbha I Aquarius	Feb 13–Mar 12	Jan 20–Feb 18
Meena I Pisces	Mar 13–Apr 12	Feb 19–Mar 20

charts

CHARTS

A Jyotish chart, or birth horoscope, is a representation of the planetary positions in relationship to the earth at the time of one's birth (date, time and place).

It shows which zodiac sign (rashi) is rising at the eastern horizon and in which signs the planets are placed in the sky. These divisions (houses or bhava) also correspond to the various areas of life they inhabit. This interconnection of planets and other elements of the horoscope (houses and signs) form a symbolic framework that reflects one's life in depth. The positions of the planets indicate which laws of nature were in effect at the time of birth.

There are two types of charts used: Northern India and Southern India style.

In the Northern chart the reading is counter clockwise, from right to left. The houses stay fixed and the signs rotate according to the rising sign.

NORTHERN INDIA CHART

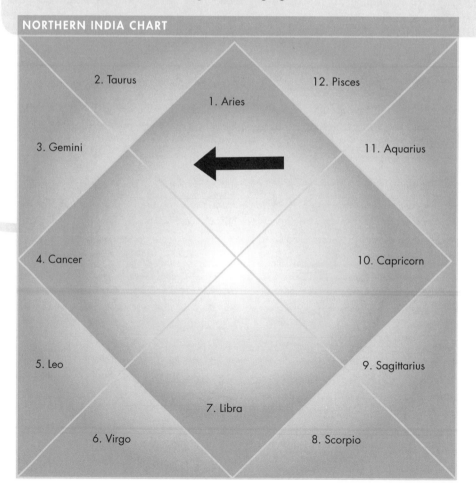

charts

CHARTS

In the Southern chart the reading is clockwise, from left to right.
The signs stay fixed and the houses move.

SOUTHERN INDIA CHART

12. Pisces	1. Aries	2. Taurus	3. Gemini
11. Aquarius			4. Cancer
10. Capricorn			5. Leo
9. Sagittarius	8. Scorpio	7. Libra	6. Virgo

Rashis

WHAT ARE RASHIS?
Signs or constellations

Rashis or signs are the division of the Zodiac in twelve equal parts of 30 degrees each. There are twelve signs and each one has its own characteristics. They influence and determine how the planets act, depending upon their strength, weakness, or neutrality. Each sign has a planet ruler, and also relates to a dosha and to a specific area of the physical body. The signs are divided into two groups:

1. By element: fire, earth, air, water

2. By quality: movable (cardinal), fixed, dual (mutable)

Pisces **Jupiter** *Kapha*	**Aries** **Mars** *Pitta*	**Taurus** **Venus** *Kapha*	**Gemini** **Mercury** *Vata*
Feet/lymphatic system	*Head*	*Face/throat/vocal chords/neck*	*Chest/shoulders/ arms/hands*
Water/Dual	*Fire/Movable*	*Earth/Fixed*	*Air/Dual*
Aquarius **Saturn** *Vata*			**Cancer** **Moon** *Kapha*
Legs/calves/ankles			*Chest/heart/ stomach/breasts*
Air/Fixed			*Water/Movable*
Capricorn **Saturn** *Pitta*			**Leo** **Sun** *Pitta*
Knees/bones/joints			*Abdomen (upper)/ circulation/stomach*
Earth/Movable			*Fire/Fixed*
Sagittarius **Jupiter** *Pitta/Kapha*	**Scorpio** **Mars** *Kapha/Pitta*	**Libra** **Venus** *Vata*	**Virgo** **Mercury** *Vata*
Thighs/hips	*Genitals/bladder/ rectum*	*Abdomen/kidneys/ reprod. organs*	*Abdomen (mid./ lower)/intestines*
Fire/Dual	*Water/Fixed*	*Air/Movable*	*Earth/Dual*

Grahas

GRAHAS
Planets

The planets are divided into two groups of natural malefic and natural benefic. They are also associated with a dosha, dhatu, element, day of the week, gem and deities. They can be debilitated or exalted, or aspected. They are divided into planetary camps (friend, enemy, and neutral) and have a house where the planet shows strength.

GRAHAS

Planet	Sun	Moon	Mars	Mercury	Jupiter
Dosha	P	K/V	P	VPK	K
Dhatu	Rakta	Rasa	Mansa	Majja	Meda
Element	Fire	Water	Fire	Earth	Earth/Water
Exalted in	Aries	Taurus	Aries/Capricorn	Virgo	Cancer
Debilitated in	Libra	Scorpio	Cancer	Pisces	Capricorn
Aspect	7	7	4/7/8	7	5/7/9
Friends	Mo/Ma/Ju	Sun, Me	Su/Mo/Ju	Su/Ve	Su/Mo/Ma
Enemies	Ve/Sa	None	Me	Mo	Me/Ve
Group	Malefic	Benefic (waxing)	Malefic	Benefic/Malefic	Benefic
House Strength	10	4	10	1	1
Day	Sunday	Monday	Tuesday	Wednesday	Thursday
Gem	Ruby	Pearl	Red coral	Emerald	Yellow Saphire
Deities	Agni/Shiva	Shakti/Parvarti	Skanda/Bhumi	Vishnu	Ganesh/Indra

GRAHAS

Planet	Venus	Saturn	Rahu	Ketu
Dosha	K/V	V	V	P
Dhatu	Shukra	Asthi	–	–
Element	Water	Air	–	–
Exalted in	Pisces	Libra	–	–
Debilitated in	Virgo	Aries	–	–
Aspect	7	3/7/10	–	–
Friends	Me/Sa	Me/Ve	–	–
Enemies	Su/Mo	Su/Mo/Ma	–	–
Group	Benefic	Malefic	–	–
House Strength	4	7	10	12
Day	Friday	Saturday	–	–
Gem	Diamond	Blue sapphire	Gomed	Cat's eye
Deities	Lakshmi	Brahma	Durga	Ganesh

V – Vata   P – Pitta   K – Kapha

Bhavas

BHAVAS
Houses

The Vedic chart is divided into 12 houses wherein the planets and signs are positioned. Each house reflects all different areas of life (internal and external). The houses are always determined based on the lagna, which is always the first house, regardless of the sign.

BHAGYA	KEYWORD	POSITION	GOAL/PLANET	BODY PART
1. Tanu	Self, body	Angular/trinal	Dharma/Aries	Head, body in general
2. Dhana	Material possessions	Maraka	Artha/Taurus	Face, mouth, throat
3. Sahaja	Growth, determination	Upachaya	Kama/Gemini	Ears, arms, neck
4. Matru	Happiness, feelings	Angular	Moksha/Cancer	Thorax, lungs, heart
5. Putra	Destiny, children	Trinal	Dharma/Leo	Heart, upper abdomen
6. Ripu	Service, struggles	Upachaya/dusthana	Artha/Virgo	Large intestines, kidney
7. Kalatra	Partnership	Angular/maraka	Kama/ Libra	Lower abdomen
8. Ayu	Longevity, health	Upachaya/dusthana	Moksha/Scorpio	Genitals, anus
9. Baghya	Knowledge, luck	Trinal	Dharma/Sagittarius	Hips, thighs
10. Karma	Career, vocation	Angular/upachaya	Artha/Capricorn	Knees
11. Labha	Gains, profits	Upachaya	Kama/Aquarius	Legs, ankles, calves
12. Moksha	Enlightenment, loss	Dusthana	Dharma/Pisces	Feet

Dashas and Gochara

DASHAS
Planetary Periods

The dashas are the periods that each planet rules. The dashas bring out the quality of the planets and dictates the conditions that one experiences at different stages in life.

PLANET	YEARS
Ketu	7
Venus	20
Sun	6
Moon	10
Mars	7
Rahu	18
Jupiter	16
Saturn	19
Mercury	17

GOCHARA
Planetary Transits

Gochara or transit is the movement of grahas or planets over the signs in the natal chart. The grahas transits have different durations and will exert less or greater influence depending on the conjunction with a planet in the natal chart. Transits should be evaluated from the house where the moon and lagna are placed.

PLANET	DURATION
Sun	One month
Moon	Two and quarter days
Mars	One and half months
Mercury	Three weeks
Jupiter	13 months
Venus	One month
Saturn	Two and half years
Rahu	One and half years
Ketu	One and half years

vedic architecture | vaastu

THE SCIENCE OF VAASTU
Vastu means dwelling or site.

Vastu is the ancient Indian science of architecture and design. Originated in the Vedas, Vastu science emphasizes the importance of following natures' rhythm and principles to achieve balance and harmony in construction of buildings and interior design. Vastu philosophy honors the five basic elements (air, fire, water, earth and space); along with nature and self. The proper alignment of these elements will create a harmonious and positive environment and well-being.

BASIC PRINCIPLES

Vastu provides a set of basic principles based on spatial directions, elevations, height, and weight; this can be applied in practical ways. The spatial directions are related to the five elements, doshas, planets and the significance of their qualities.

VAASTU PURUSHA MANDALA

The combination of Ayurvedic knowledge and Vaastu Purusha mandala helps in the planning of a house in a manner that energy flows, creating a sense of harmony. This chart is a guide to find success in applying Vaastu principles.

Vaastu purusha lies facing down with his head placed towards Northeast, which is the direction of wisdom and spirituality. The right side lies on the East and South and the left side lies on the West and North.

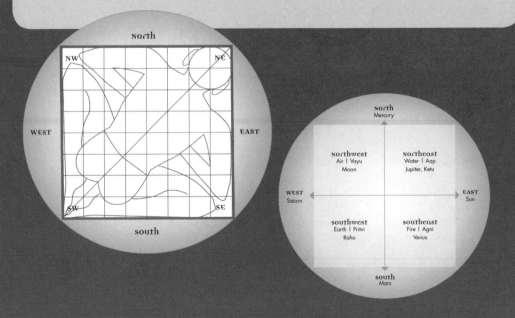

vaastu principles

BASIC APPLICATIONS OF VAASTU

EXAMPLES FOR CONSTRUCTION OR SITE

Plots/sites in Southwest, South and West directions are more advantageous than others.

Rectangular or square shapes are more advisable.

North should be lower than South, so the site should be sloping towards North.

It is advisable to have equal open space on all four sides.

South and West should have less open space and be at a higher elevation.

ENTRANCE

The most beneficial entrances to the house are those in the Northeast, East or North directions.
The width of the door should be half of its height. Square and automatic doors should be avoided.

LIVING ROOM

The best locations are North, Northeast, East or West directions. The center area of a living room (Brahma sthan) should be free of obstructions such as pillars, fixtures, or staircases.

BEDROOM

It can be located in any quadrant except Southeast direction.

KIDS' BEDROOM

Northwest is recommended, avoid Southeast and Southwest.

GUEST BEDROOM

It is best if located in Northwest or Northeast directions.

STUDY ROOM

All directions are good except Northwest. It is best to sit facing East or North.

KITCHEN

The most ideal location is the Southeast direction.

BATHROOM

Northwest, West or South direction are recommended.

SLEEP

Never sleep with the head in the North quadrant; all other directions are positive.

music | gandharva veda

MUSIC THERAPY

Gandharva Veda is Upaveda, a branch of Vedic literature. It is the ancient science of sound, music and melodies. The universe (one song or verse) has different rhythms and frequencies at every level of creation. From dawn to dusk, fall to spring and at different stages of life, Gandharva Veda is nothing but the arrangement of these primordial frequencies of nature. By creating melodies and musical compositions, musical instruments have a calming and harmonizing effect on the physiology.

The seven musical notes are directly related with the seven chakras and do have a regulatory effect on the pranic body. There are different Ragas and melodies that synchronize with different times of the day and night, and have a balancing effect on Vata, Pitta and Kapha. Playing and listening to string, air instruments and drums affect Vata, Pitta and Kapha respectively.

DOSHA	SOUND	INSTRUMENT
VATA	Soothing, nourishing, calming music	Harmonium, piano
PITTA	Cooler, light	Flute, clarinet
KAPHA	Stimulating	Drums, bongo, conga

CHAKRA	SOUND (SWAR)	RAAG	INSTRUMENT
Mooladhara	"Sa"	Bilawal	Shehenai
Swadishthana	Komal "Re"	Todi	Veena
Manipura	Komal "Ga"	Bhatiyar	Santoor
Anahata	Shudda "Ma"	Bhairava	Tabla-Drums
Vishuddha	"Pa"	Jay-Jayawanti	Flute
Ajna	Komal "Dha"	Bageshri	Sarod
Sahasrara	"Ni"	Darbari	Sitar

References

Charaka Samhita, Ashtang Hriday.

Cox, Kathleen. The Power of Vastu Living.
New York, NY: Fireside Publishing, 2002

Frawley, Dr. David. Ayurvedic Healing, A Comprehensive Guide.
Twin Lakes, Wisconsin; Lotus Press, 2000

Frawley, Dr. David; Ranade, Dr. Subhash and Lele, Dr. Avinash.
Ayurveda and Marma Therapy
Twin Lakes, Wisconsin; Lotus Press, 2000

Frawley, Dr. David. Yoga and Ayurveda.
Twin Lakes, Wisconsin; Lotus Press, 1999

Frawley, Dr. David and Kozac, Sandra. Yoga for your Type.
Twin Lakes, Wisconsin; Lotus Press, 2007

Frawley, Dr. David and Lad, Dr. Vasant. The Yoga of Herbs.
Twin Lakes, Wisconsin; Lotus Press, 2000

Kerala Ayurveda Academy. Lessons 101-109. Foster City, CA, 2009

Lad, Dr. Vasant. Ayurveda, The Science of Self-Healing.
Twin Lakes, Wisconsin; Lotus Press, 1984

Lad, Dr. Vasant. Textbook of Ayurveda, Fundamental Principles, Volume 1.
Albuquerque. NM: Ayurvedic Press, 2002

Lad, Dr. Vasant. The Complete Book of Ayurvedic Home Remedies.
New York, NY; Three Rivers Press, 1999

Levacy, William R. Beneath a Vedic Sky.
Ontario, CA; Hay House, Inc., 1999

Sarsvati, Satyananda. Asan, Pranayam, Mudra, Bandha.
Yoga Publications Trust, Munger, Bihar, India, 2008

Tirtha, Swami Sadashiva. The Ayurveda Encyclopedia.
Bayville, NY; Ayurvedic Holistic Center Press, 1998

about the authors

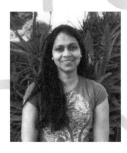

Dr. Manisha has an extensive background in Ayurveda. She is the Director of the Ayurvedic Healing Clinic in Santa Cruz, CA. Currently, she is a faculty member at Mount Madonna College of Ayurveda and Kerala Ayurveda Academy.

Dr. Manisha's credentials are as follows:

B.A.M.S. (Bachelor of Ayurvedic Medicine & Surgery), Pune University 1989

Diplomate Yoga & Ayurveda, Tilak Maharashtra University, 1987

Yoga Teacher Certification, Kaivalyadham University, 1984

N.D. at Indian College of Naturopathy, Nasik, 1992

Licensed Esthetician, Hawaii, 2005

Licensed Massage Therapist, Hawaii 2004

Professor at Maharishi European Research University, 1994-1999, Netherlands

Professor at Maharishi College of Vedic Medicine, 1999-2002, Fairfield, IA

Ayurveda Physician at Kauai Center for Holistic Medicine, 2003-2007, Hawaii

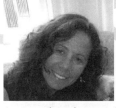

Ana Cristina is an Ayurvedic Wellness Counselor and has been involved in the complementary health field for many years. Ana is also a professional Graphic Designer.

Ana's credentials are as follows:

B.A. in Communication Design, UniverCidade University, Rio, Brazil, 1984

M.S. in Communication Design, Pratt Institute, New York City, 1988

Dl. Hom., British Institute of Homeopathy, CA, 2001

A.W.C., Ayurvedic Wellness Counselor, Kerala Ayurveda Academy, CA, 2010

C.M.T., Certified Massage Therapist, South Bay Massage College, CA, 2010